Educators' Stories of Creating Enduring Change

ENHANCING THE PROFESSIONAL CULTURE OF ACADEMIC HEALTH SCIENCE CENTERS

Edited by

LINDA A. HEADRICK, MD, MS
Helen Mae Spiese Distinguished Faculty Scholar
Senior Associate Dean for Education and Professor of Medicine
School of Medicine, University of Missouri
Columbia, MO, USA

and

DEBRA K. LITZELMAN, MA, MD
Professor of Medicine and Associate Dean for Research in Medical Education
Indiana University School of Medicine
Indianapolis, IN, USA

Associate Editors

ANN H. COTTINGHAM, MAR, MA
Director, Dean's Office for Research in Medical Education,
Indiana University School of Medicine

and

JANE L. MANDEL, BA
Business Technology Analyst, University of Missouri School of Medicine

Foreword by
DAVID C. LEACH, MD

CULTURE, CONTEXT AND QUALITY IN HEALTH SCIENCES
RESEARCH, EDUCATION, LEADERSHIP AND PATIENT CARE

Series Editors
THOMAS S. INUI AND RICHARD M. FRANKEL

Radcliffe Publishing
London • New York

Radcliffe Publishing Ltd
33–41 Dallington Street
London
EC1V 0BB
United Kingdom

www.radcliffehealth.com

British Library Cataloguing in Publication Data

A catalogue record for this book is available from the British Library.

ISBN-13: 978 184619 531 0

Typeset by Darkriver Design, Auckland, New Zealand

Contents

Contents

Foreword

Stories move in circles, not in straight lines. So it helps if you listen in circles. There are stories inside stories and stories between stories, and finding your way through them is as easy and as hard as finding your way home. And part of the finding is the getting lost. And when you're lost, you start to look around and to listen.
— Albert Greenberg, Corey Fischer, and Naomi Newman[1]

THAT WHICH USED TO BE CALLED CONTINUING EDUCATION IS increasingly being referred to as professional formation. The word education evokes thinking about something outside that is brought in, something that is abstract and detached from particular context and yet offers a guide to life. The word formation gets us closer to the truth; it describes a shaping experience, it suggests that we are shaped by context; it invites thinking about internal as well as external shaping forces, it provokes deep attention to context. Professional formation begins in experience and is mostly dependent on two things: people and the relationships they have with one another. Think back to your own formative experiences – particular patients, colleagues from the various professions that you have worked with, others who while not labeled professional were formative to those around them, and recall the stories that you constructed based on your experiences and then told and retold in an attempt to make sense of the world. This book is about such stories. It brings together stories, diverse stories reflecting different journeys toward the same end: attending to professional formation for the purpose of improving patient care. Stories don't go in straight lines. It is easy to get lost on this journey and, "when you're lost, you start to look around and to listen."[1] This book invites the reader to look around and to listen, to develop the habit of listening and seeing the various sets of people and their relationships in your own particular contexts and to recognize the communities on your particular journey toward attending to those people and relationships in ways that improve patient care.

As I read the stories in this book and reflected on my own experiences, I found that I had taken some detours on my journey. My detours included compartmentalizing education; refining educational outcome measures while ignoring patient outcomes; focusing on one health profession while ignoring others; focusing on individuals, programs, or systems without appreciating the effects each has on the others. Yet, at least in my case, the detour became part of the journey. For me, attending to professional formation for the purpose of improving patient care was not simply a matter of going from here to there. It was, in fact, an inner journey, and it began by trying to improve myself. About 25 years ago, while still at the Henry Ford Health System, I took a course offered by Paul Batalden: his Quality 101 course. His first assignment was for everyone in the class to attempt to improve something about themselves. I chose to try to shorten my response time to clinical phone calls. Like many quality improvement efforts this one began in experience and in frustration with experience – I found being swamped by phone messages and not being able to respond quickly frustrating. I began by gathering data, understanding the causes of variation in response time, changing my behavior, and monitoring the results. I learned a tremendous amount about myself and about my practice. The gaps between ideal and real went beyond returning phone calls. I found that while being more conscious about my experiences and those of my patients and reflecting on these experiences was necessary, it was not sufficient. I needed a community as well. I needed both time alone to develop my reflections and time in community to share them and to see how well they held up under scrutiny. This metareflection led to two new tasks: how to develop quality reflection time for myself and how to structure time in community for conversations about improvement. At this point I got lost. I had a very busy practice and lots of administrative duties; I could not see how I could both practice and improve my practice at the same time. It took time to gather data, to plan an intervention, to study the effect of the intervention, and to share and study what I was doing. It was much easier to just continue with my habits – or so I thought.

Noticing frustrations was helpful; I began to harvest them. At that point I was heavily engaged with teaching residents and they could frequently be overheard saying: "It's really weird how they do things around here." When I inquired into what they were noticing I found that residents knew a tremendous amount about the systems in which they worked and learned but that they felt unempowered to change the context of their work. The things they were noticing were associated with both the quality of patient care and the quality of life of all who work in the system. The things they were noticing came about because of decisions, habits, and policies that were generated from the micro-, meso-, and macrosystems in which they worked and learned and sometimes by national policies. Often they came about because of unexamined assumptions about the expectations of the various parties. Examining these assumptions required a level of civility that would support open, honest dialogue – a level of civility that was not uniform across all of the involved systems. The task was daunting. I got lost again. Taking residents seriously was going to cause a social revolution. As a child of the sixties, revolutions appealed to me, but this seemed too much. Fortunately, by then I had discovered Parker Palmer, who taught me that revolutions do not originate in hate or anger, but rather in love: "They occur when you love your (practice, institution, profession, country, . . .) so much that you won't let it fall to its most degraded state" (Parker J. Palmer, personal communication, May 5, 2001). Improvement became a moral issue driven by love – and here I was well into middle age – it was invigorating. Furthermore, this framing became such an attractor that my earlier dilemma of how to find the right community was resolved – everybody wanted to improve their profession and wanted to improve patient care.

Each person has an improvement story to tell. This book captures some good ones. Each of these authors is a sophisticated observer and truthteller. They have told us what they noticed, how they made sense of what they noticed, and how they took action to improve professional formation and patient care. The result is a gift. There are victories (small and large), frustrations, lessons, and mostly the realization that there is an emerging community of people interested in such things. It turns out that there are lots of people interested in professional formation. Why should they or anyone pay attention to professional formation, why not just take care of patients and go home? These authors know that professional formation and the quality of patient care are inextricably linked. You cannot learn good patient care habits in a system that cannot reliably deliver good patient care, and you cannot deliver good patient care without attending to professional formation. Good patient care and good learning both require an ecology that is nourishing and which will support life.

I would like to do an analysis of the DNA of each of the authors and their teams – perhaps there is an "improvement gene" that drives each one of them. Most of us look around and say: "It's really weird how they do things around here," and call it a day. These innovators seem genetically incapable of supporting a status quo that delivers less than optimal care for patients, and they seem to know at some level that health professional formation is the key to fixing the "weird things." We can learn much from their work and their stories.

David C. Leach, MD
Asheville, North Carolina
April 2013

Reference

1. Greenberg A, Fischer C, Newman N. *Coming From A Great Distance*. Unpublished play performed at Traveling Jewish Theater, San Francisco. 1979.

Preface

This book will present a web of stories about people whose work in medical education has touched the lives of others in important ways. The intended impact is to deepen the reader's self-awareness, generating a realization of the individual's capacity for creating enduring change, helping others to be the best they can be. The reader says, "I can do that, too."

—Notes from "Finding the thread: three days in Oxford"[1]

WE WOULD LIKE TO SHARE OUR STORY OF HOW WE CONCEIVED OF AND gave birth to this education volume in the Culture, Context and Quality in Health Sciences Research, Education, Leadership and Patient Care series. Linda and Deb were both honored to be approached by Tom Inui who asked if we would serve as coeditors of this volume in the Inui and Frankel Radcliffe series. An undeniable treat was the opportunity to have all the volume editors gather at the Radcliffe Publishing offices in Oxford where the ideas and plans for all volumes in the series were conceived. As a collective group, we agreed to gather and tell stories about how individuals made major impacts in their respective Academic Health Science Centers (AHSCs) working with a larger network of individuals. We wanted to share their stories about how they built and disseminated programs that mutually influenced their own personal growth while simultaneously influencing the culture in which they worked. We wanted these stories to serve as an inspiration to our readers. With this framework in mind, Linda and I also met separately while at Oxford to plan the *who, what, why, and how* for the education volume. Back in the United States, we were fortunate to be joined by our associate editors, Ann Cottingham and Jane Mandel, who were instrumental in helping move our ideas to reality.

Who
. . . .

From our own vantage points as education administrators, curriculum innovators, and health professional educators, we identified education innovators who have made an impact on learners, teachers, and the cultures of AHSCs at a national and even international level. It was immediately clear that because of space limitations we would not be able to include many wonderful education innovators who have had a major impact. However, we made every effort to include authors from large, small, public, and private AHSCs as well as from individuals who built a new medical school and residency training programs at an Indiana University sister medical school in Kenya where Deb has served as an educational consultant-partner. Many of the programs built by the authors arose from grassroots efforts; however, others received start-up funds from foundations such as the Macy Foundation, the Robert Wood Johnson Foundation, and the Fetzer Institute.

What

This book is a web of stories about people whose work in health professions education has touched the lives of others in important ways. Each chapter is told from the point of view of an education innovator and is supplemented by short reflections from individuals whose lives have been changed as a result of that work. Our intent is for the full story of each chapter to be told from the voices of a *network*, a web of interconnected individuals affected in different ways by the innovation. Innovative education programs described in the chapters are programs that have had a transformative impact on the program participants, the organizational environments or professional cultures associated with the program, and health professional education itself. The closing chapter includes the results of appreciative inquiry interviews with chapter authors. The intended impact of this volume is to generate a deeper understanding of individual capacity for creating enduring change.

In thinking about the success stories to be told by these individuals, we chose to focus on the process of innovation that in most cases evolved over decades of work (in one case over 6 decades, as one of our authors turns 96 soon!). Since the process of innovation evolves and moves through various phases from conceptualization, to implementation, to evaluation, to dissemination, we did not attempt to organize chapters into tidy, traditional education categories such as curriculum development, assessment and evaluation, faculty development, and dissemination. However, readers will find numerous examples of all of these within the stories.

Why

We wanted to inspire other educators to live their dreams by following in the footsteps of a group of leaders in health professional education. By helping the authors tell their stories, we wanted the readers to experience their deep commitment – actually, it was more like a deep conviction – to realizing their vision of ways to improve health professional education and the learning environments. We asked these education leaders to write "their stories" and lace their professional journeys with stories from those whom they have influenced along the way. In the end, our goal was to have a collection of librettos that would inspire readers to say, "I can do that!"

- *I can* create a course so wonderful that students and teachers petition to make it a required course, or
- *I can* create a new curriculum that would allow interprofessional colleagues to learn and grow together in preparation for practicing in relational team-based environments, or
- *I can* create a faculty development program so influential that participants send their colleagues and they come back to contribute as teachers, or
- *I can* bring people together in ways to generate new conversations, new relationships, new patterns of behavior, with a resultant new culture, or
- *I can* do something completely new that makes a significant contribution to health professional education.

How

Once engaged, we asked authors to tell the story from their personal point of view. We wanted to hear about their hopes and dreams. We wanted to find out about who they thought would benefit from their work. We wanted to know what they had learned along the way; what was most surprising, satisfying, and challenging. We asked them to look back and reflect about what had changed as a result of their work including the effect on the professional culture at their own and other AHSCs. We asked them to share their dreams for the future of their work. Finally, we asked the authors to identify individuals who felt the impact of their work and to invite them to provide their personal reflections related to key elements described in the chapter body. We then worked with the authors to help integrate the stories-within-the-story in order to weave the intricate web of relationships involved in the process of successful education innovation.

Appreciative Inquiry Interviews

Lastly, we conducted interviews of all the primary authors using an appreciative inquiry interview method.[2] We conducted the interviews using a well-standardized set of appreciative inquiry questions including the following.

- Please think of an incident, an occasion, or a circumstance in which you have felt successful, just like yourself and really effective in your role as an education innovator. Please tell me the story of that occasion. It need not be a monumental success. It could be a recent event or one from the distant past. The right one to report is the first one that comes to your mind!
- After listening to the story and asking for any clarifications, the interview asks three additional probes:
  - What did you bring to this situation to allow this success to materialize?
  - I notice there are other people in the story – what did they contribute to this success?
  - Was there something about the organizational environment, policies, or resources that supported this success?

The interviews lasted from 30 to 60 minutes. With permission from the interviewees, the interviews were recorded and later transcribed. We then read all the transcripts and through thematic analysis identified the prominent content described in our final chapter.

In the interviews, these leaders' character traits and styles – passion, vision, risk taking, open-mindedness, curiosity, belief in others and teamwork, and tenacity – emerged. The ability of these individuals to translate their core values and principles into local, national, and international programs stood out. These education innovators created a legacy by building a community of like-minded individuals and helped empower others to spread and sustain the work over time. Importantly, the chapter authors emerged as role models who inspired their colleagues and the next generation of health care professional educators to believe that positive change in the learning environments of AHSCs is possible – to say "I *can* do that."

Debra K. Litzelman, Linda A. Headrick,
and Ann H. Cottingham
April 2013

References

1. Beyt G. Finding the thread: three days in Oxford. 2010. Unpublished booklet by one of the Culture, Context and Quality in Health Sciences Research, Education, Leadership and Patient Care series volume editors.
2. Cooperrider DL, Srivastva S. Appreciative inquiry in organizational life. *Res Organ Change Dev.* 1987; **1**: 129–69.

List of Contributors

Armstrong, Elizabeth G., PhD, is the Director of the Harvard Macy Institute, a Clinical Professor in Pediatrics at Harvard Medical School, and an adjunct Professor at the Massachusetts General Hospital Institute of Health Professions. Dr. Armstrong's professional focus is on the development, implementation, and evaluation of educational programs across the continuum of health care professions. She serves on the Editorial Board of Academic Medicine and on the Board of Trustees of the F. W. Olin College of Engineering. She is recognized internationally for her contributions to advances in health care education and received an Honorary Doctor of Medicine from Lund University. She holds degrees from Cornell University, Harvard University, and Boston College.

Ayuo, Paul O., MBChB, MMed, Dip & MSc, has been the dean of Moi University School of Medicine since August 2009 and is an associate Professor of Medicine in the Department of Internal Medicine. Professor Ayuo joined Moi University in 1991 and has held various portfolios in the school including chairing the committees charged with overseeing the implementation and/or development of undergraduate and graduate curricula at the school. In addition, Professor Ayuo was the second head of the Department of Internal Medicine from 1994 to 2000. Professor Ayuo is a physician with an interest in health professionals' education, gastroenterology, and public health.

Baldwin, Jr., DeWitt C., MD, ScD(hon), DHL(hon), is a pediatrician, family physician, and psychiatrist who has served on the faculties of eight medical schools, two dental schools, three graduate schools, and two schools of social work. His career is devoted to advancing humanism, primary care, the behavioral and social sciences, and interprofessional education and practice in health care. Since retiring from the presidency of Earlham College in Richmond, Indiana, in 1984, he has resumed a distinguished career in medical and interprofessional education and research – initially, at the American Medical Association, and more recently with the Accreditation Council for Graduate Medical Education.

Barsion, Sylvia, PhD, is an educator and researcher specializing in assessment of learning outcomes. As president of SJB Evaluation & Research Consultants LLC, she has worked with the Harvard Macy Institute, Massachusetts Institute of Technology, and Northeastern University as well as with numerous nonprofit organizations. Dr. Barsion has taught graduate courses in Research Design and Outcomes Measurement. She earned her doctorate in Educational Research, Measurement and Evaluation at Boston College.

Branch, Jr., William T., MD, MACP, served as Director of the Division of General Internal Medicine (1995–2012) and is the Carter Smith Sr. Professor of Medicine, in the Department of Medicine, Emory University School of Medicine. Prior to that, Dr. Branch was Associate Professor of Medicine and Director of the Third-Year Patient-Doctor Relationship Course at Harvard Medical School and Director of the Primary Care Residency Program at Brigham and Women's Hospital. Dr. Branch's career is focused on medical education, humanism in medicine, and patient-doctor communication.

Cottingham, Ann H., MAR, MA, is the Director of the Dean's Office for Research in Medical Education and has worked in the field of medical education for over 10 years, developing curricula and furthering research in the areas of clinical ethics, professionalism, physician-patient relationships, shared decision making, and communication around end-of-life care. She served as a co-investigator and member of the leadership team for the Indiana University School of Medicine Relationship-Centered Care Initiative designed to study the impact of organizational change strategies on the professional and educational culture of Indiana University School of Medicine/Indiana University Health System.

Einterz, Robert M., MD, is the director of the Indiana University Center for Global Health and a practicing general internist. His career is focused on developing partnerships among academic health centers and delivering health care services to underserved populations in Indianapolis and western Kenya.

Frankel, Richard M., PhD, is a Professor of Medicine and Geriatrics and the Director of the Mary Margaret Walter Center for Palliative Care Research and Education at Melvin and Bren Simon Cancer Center, Indiana University School of Medicine. He is also the Associate Director of the Center for Implementing Evidence-Based Practice at the Richard L. Roudebush Veteran's Administration Medical Center. He is a qualitative health researcher whose career has been focused on relationship-centered communication and its effect(s) on a variety of health care and organizational outcomes.

Headrick, Linda A., MD, MS, is Helen Mae Spiese Distinguished Faculty Scholar, Senior Associate Dean for Education, and Professor of Medicine at the School of Medicine, University of Missouri in Columbia, Missouri. Her academic work has focused on quality improvement in health care and health professional education, with an emphasis on preparing new health professionals to improve care as part of their daily practice. Dr. Headrick received her AB in Chemistry at the University of Missouri-Columbia, MD at Stanford University, and MS in Epidemiology and Biostatistics at Case Western Reserve University.

Holmboe, Eric, MD, FACP, FRCP, currently serves as Chief Medical Officer and Senior Vice President at the American Board of Internal Medicine. A board-certified physician in internal medicine, Dr. Holmboe received his medical degree from the University of Rochester and completed his residency and chief residency at Yale-New Haven Hospital. He completed the Robert Wood Johnson Clinical Scholars Fellowship Program at Yale University.

Inui, Thomas S., ScM, MD, MACP, is Joe and Sarah Ellen Mamlin Professor of Global Health Research and the Director of Research, Indiana University Center for Global Health, as well as Senior Investigator in the Regenstrief Institute, Inc. Dr. Inui's special emphases in teaching and research have included physician-patient communication, health promotion and disease prevention, chronic disease management, the social context of medicine, and medical humanities.

Iobst, William, MD, is Vice President of Academic Affairs at the American Board of Internal Medicine. In this capacity, Dr. Iobst develops outreach activities with internal medicine residency and fellowship training programs as well as faculty development programs addressing competency-based medical education. He also works with the American Board of Internal Medicine's research team to develop new and better assessment methodologies for competency evaluation.

Jackson, Marcy, MSW, MPH, is cofounder and Senior Fellow for the Center for Courage and Renewal. She was Co-Director of the Center for 13 years. Marcy leads the Center for Courage and Renewal's Facilitator Preparation Program and supports the ongoing development of 200 facilitators in the United States, Canada, and Australia. She has been facilitating Courage and Renewal retreats since 1996 with people from a variety of backgrounds and professions. Previously, Marcy worked extensively with individuals, groups, and families as a child and family therapist, grief counselor, and group facilitator.

Leach, David C., MD, is the retired Chief Executive Officer of the Accreditation Council for Graduate Medical Education. His career focused on teaching and the practice of medicine. He is particularly interested in graduate medical education, how physicians acquire competence, and in the role of chaordic organizations in creating an ecology that supports sets of relationships more apt to support the formation of good physicians. He has received honorary degrees from five medical schools. He is a member of the Gold Humanism Honorary Society and is the 2007 recipient of the Abraham Flexner Award for Distinguished Service to Medical Education.

Litzelman, Debra K., MA, MD, is Professor of Medicine and Associate Dean for Research in Medical Education at the Indiana University School of Medicine (IUSM). As Associate Dean for Medical Education and Curricular Affairs from 2002 to 2011, she helped develop, implement and assess an innovative competency-based curriculum for the IUSM. Dr. Litzelman served as the Co-Principal Investigator on the Relationship-Centered Care Initiative directed at influencing and studying the impact of organizational change strategies on the IUSM's professional learning environment. Her research focuses on the impact of interventions customized to prepare health care providers for their roles in team-based, relational, and collaborative models of care.

Mengech, Haroun, MB, ChB, DPM, MRCPsych, MD, MBS, EBS, is a Professor of Mental Health in the College of Health Sciences, School of Medicine, Moi University. He is the previous Director of Moi Teaching and Referral Hospital and the founding Dean of the second Medical School in Kenya in 1988. Prof. Mengech was credited for introducing Innovative Medical Education in Kenya, if not in sub-Saharan Africa. He went on to build the Moi Teaching and Referral Hospital as a Center of Excellence in Learning, Clinical Care and Research. He holds honors from the Kenyan Government, Linkoping University, and Maastricht University, among others.

Moore, Shirley M., RN, PhD, FAAN, is the Edward J. and Louise Mellon Professor of Nursing and Associate Dean for Research, Case Western Reserve University, Cleveland, Ohio. She is a past President of the Academy for Healthcare Improvement and is on the leadership team of the national Quality and Safety Education for Nurses (QSEN) project. She is currently leading the integration of nurse scholars into the Veterans Affairs National Quality Scholars Fellowship Program. She also is conducting National Institutes of Health-funded studies testing a process improvement approach to health behavior change with patients.

Palmer, Parker J., PhD, is an independent writer, speaker, and activist who focuses on issues in education, community, leadership, spirituality, and social change. He is founder and Senior Partner of the Center for Courage and Renewal, which oversees long-term retreat programs for people in the serving professions. Palmer has authored nine books, including *Healing the Heart of Democracy*, *The Courage to Teach*, *A Hidden Wholeness*, and *Let Your Life Speak*. He holds a PhD in sociology from the University of California at Berkeley as well as 11 honorary doctorates.

Quigley, Fran, MA, JD, is Clinical Professor of Law and director of the Health and Human Rights Clinic at Indiana University Robert H. McKinney School of Law. He is currently writing a book about human rights in Haiti.

Skeff, Kelley M., MD, PhD, is the Co-Director of the Stanford Faculty Development Center for Medical Teachers, and is the Vice-Chair for Education and Professor of Medicine in the Department of Medicine at Stanford University. He is Master of the American College of Physicians (ACP), an ACP Regent, and was the residency program director in internal medicine at Stanford for 2 decades. Dr. Skeff's career has been focused on the improvement of medical education with a special focus on faculty development.

Smith, Dale, BA, BJ, is a freelance writer and editor whose clients are university faculty members in disciplines including medicine, nursing, sociology, and physical therapy. During the past 2 decades, Smith has edited grant applications, articles, dissertations, and books. He has contributed editing expertise to numerous National Institutes of Health proposals and to journal articles appearing in the *New England Journal of Medicine*, the *Journal of the American Medical Association*, and *Pediatrics*, among others. Smith also has researched and written about health care topics for experts and mass audiences.

Stratos, Georgette A., PhD, is Co-Director of the Stanford Faculty Development Center for Medical Teachers and Senior Research Scholar in the Division of General Medical Disciplines, Department of Medicine at Stanford University Medical School. Dr. Stratos holds a doctoral degree in educational psychology from the University of California, Berkeley. Her career has focused on methods of assisting medical faculty and residents to improve their teaching effectiveness.

Suchman, Anthony L., MD, MA, FAACH, is a practicing internist, health services researcher, consultant, and professor of medicine and a leading advocate of Relationship-Centered Care. His current work focuses on organizational behavior in health care – fostering leadership behavior and work environments that treat staff members in the same way we want them to treat patients and families. He has recently published his second book, *Leading Change in Healthcare* (coauthored with David Sluyter and Penny Williamson), which presents principles and case studies in relationship-centered administration. He directs the Healthcare Consultancy at the McArdle Ramerman Center in Rochester, New York.

Viggiano, Thomas R., MD, MEd, is Associate Dean for Faculty Affairs in Mayo Medical School and Director, Office of Innovation and Scholarship, College of Medicine, Mayo Clinic. He is also the Barbara Woodward Lips Professor, and Professor of Medical Education and Medicine, College of Medicine, Mayo Clinic. Dr. Viggiano is board certified in internal medicine, gastroenterology, and geriatric medicine and specializes in therapeutic endoscopy. He has served on and chaired numerous national and international boards and executive committees for medical education. Dr. Viggiano has published and delivered invited presentations on professionalism and leadership in medical education.

Williamson, Penelope R., ScD, is a senior consultant for Relationship-Centered Health Care, a part time Associate Professor of Medicine at The Johns Hopkins University School of Medicine and a founding facilitator for The National Center for Courage and Renewal. She facilitates personal and professional development retreat programs for leaders in health care and other serving professions, and coaches individual leaders, leadership groups, working teams, and organizations to build sustainable capacities in collaborative learning and relationship-centered practice.

Acknowledgments

THIS VOLUME COULD NOT HAVE BEEN COMPLETED WITHOUT THE substantial assistance from the two associate editors, Ann Cottingham and Jane Mandel, who shared in every phase of nurturing and birthing this volume. Ann Cottingham not only contributed as the lead author of one of the chapters and as coauthor of the Preface and our final chapter but also read, edited, and made major contributions to the content of the entire volume. Jane Mandel contributed her expertise in detailed editing and formatting. Sharree Rose, from the University of Missouri, transcribed many hours of the audiotaped appreciative inquiry interviews conducted with the authors, and Kathie Mullins, from Indiana University, assisted with creating figures and maps and other numerous administrative details. We are extremely grateful for the assistance, laughter, and encouragement provided by Ann, Jane, Sharree, and Kathie along the way. Finally, we wish to acknowledge the National Institutes of Health Office of Behavioral and Social Sciences Research and the National Institute of Arthritis and Musculoskeletal and Skin Diseases (Request for Application OD-05-001 – K07 and 5R25AR060994-02) for partial support of Deb Litzelman's and Ann Cottingham's time to create this volume.

Debra K. Litzelman and Linda A. Headrick

To my father, Hubert H. Headrick, whose life of giving to others has always inspired me.

—Linda A. Headrick

To my mother, Beryl E. Litzelman, for her ever-loving presence.

—Debra K. Litzelman

Health Care from the Inside Out

Bringing the Self of the Healer into the Practice of Medicine

An Interview with Parker J. Palmer by Marcy Jackson

In 1992, Parker J. Palmer was invited by the Fetzer Institute to develop a program of support and renewal for public school teachers. This led to a retreat series called "Courage to Teach" and, eventually, to the creation of the Center for Courage & Renewal. After this work with educators became more widely known, and after Parker published *The Courage to Teach: Exploring the Inner Landscape of a Teacher's Life*,[1] other professionals – including those in health care – expressed urgent interest in the need for such exploration in their lives and professions. In addition, the Accreditation Council for Graduate Medical Education (ACGME) launched an awards program around the key ideas in *The Courage to Teach*, and Deb Litzelman and colleagues at the Indiana University School of Medicine launched a system-wide set of initiatives and programs based on the ideas and practices that Palmer had developed in his writing and in his work with teachers in "Courage to Teach" retreats. In this chapter we trace the manifestation of these ideas in health care.

Marcy Jackson (MJ): How did you get involved in working with health care professionals and medical educators?

Parker J. Palmer (PJP): When I wrote *The Courage to Teach*[1] – or published it, in 1998 – I really wasn't thinking about health care educators. I was thinking about undergraduate education, adult education, and about K-12 [kindergarten through twelfth grade] education. And maybe a little bit about professional education. But certainly not health care education in particular. But it was because of that book, and some articles that had come out before the book, that Don Berwick at the IHI [Institute for Healthcare Improvement] called and asked if I would address the national conference of IHI in Orlando.

And what's interesting is that I don't remember whether it was his guidance or my decision or both, but in that talk I ended up talking not so much about teaching and learning – which was the main focus of the book – but about the "movement model." And in ways I hadn't anticipated, it was very illuminating for the audience because they were obviously people who were wrestling with the whole question of how do you change the health care system. And the idea of a movement for change, rather than a more top-down organizational model of change, was appealing to them.

MJ: Can you say more about the movement model?

PJP: Well, stage one of the movement model is this decision to "live divided no more." It's really about the power of human integrity. And I think what people were hearing (which is what I hoped they would hear) is that a physician who has taken the Hippocratic oath needs to reclaim his or her integrity – to live by that oath – under circumstances that are often very challenging or threatening to that oath. Then the movement model unfolds from that individual, inward decision into different forms of collective support and then outward into different avenues of institutional transformation.

So that talk, which was recorded on DVD, started getting quite a bit of circulation and led to some amazing connections and opened some doors for us in health care.

MJ: I know one of those amazing connections was with the ACGME – a connection that led to the creation of the Parker J. Palmer Courage to Teach Awards Program. How did that come about?

PJP: This is a wonderful story that has meant a lot to me. Sometime in the summer of 2000 I got a phone call in my office from a man called David Leach, MD, who introduced himself as the executive director of a national organization in Chicago called the ACGME – the Accreditation Council for Graduate Medical Education – the organization that accredits all of the medical residency programs in the United States.

David Leach said to me, "We've been reading *The Courage to Teach*[1] and watching the IHI DVD, and we know about the program that you have been doing with K-12 teachers. I've shared this with my board and with my staff and we collectively think that you folks are talking about the kind of standards that we want residency education to measure up to so that we turn out doctors who aspire to, and have the capacity to, achieve high levels of professionalism." This is their term for what I would call "humanism in medicine": the capacity of a doctor to do his or her technical work with heart in hand as it were, connecting with the patient at a human level, evoking the patient's own heart and spiritual and psychological powers of healing, as well as working with the body.

He went on to say, "We have a plan, and the plan is that every year for a decade, we will solicit nominations from our community for ten Courage to Teach award winners from ten exemplary programs. Their directors would be honored at a banquet in Chicago, and then we'll work with you to bring them together every summer in a Circle of Trust retreat so that they can deepen their understanding of [formation] principles and go back to their programs better able to implement these principles and practices. And more than that," he said, "we want to build a community of high practice, of high commitment, and high competence around humanism in medicine, so that at the end of a decade we will have created a huge conversation in our community that will allow us to change the accreditation standards so that all 8100 residency programs live up to a new norm for the doing of medicine. A norm which is not only about technical competence and knowledge base, but also about the capacity to enter humane relationships, relationships that evoke spirit and soul – relationships that help patients heal."

In about 15 minutes, this amazing man, whom I quickly understood to be brilliant, passionate, committed, and highly effective, is asking me, "Would you have any interest in doing this?" I'm sitting there, thinking, "Well, gosh, I don't know. He's one of the most remarkable people I've ever talked to, and the resources are lined up to do something that sounds amazingly worth doing. And I think in about a microsecond I screeched at him, "How soon can we begin?"

Since then, David Leach and Paul Batalden and others from the ACGME have become great personal friends and also extraordinary professional colleagues for all of us involved in this Circle of Trust work. They have shown us on a new level of institutional reality what it means to take these principles and practices into an institution like an accrediting agency – an agency that has tremendous power over the lives of lots of other institutions in this country – and to use that power for the highest good. Their goal is to help create more humane forms of medical education that don't burn people out on being doctors, that don't exhaust them and wear them down, that don't deplete their resources, but that actually enlarge their inner store of heart and soul and spirit so that they can be doctors and healers in the fullest sense of that term. It's simply been one of the most rewarding professional relationships that we've had on this journey and it's taught us a lot about the process of linking soul and role work with large-scale institutional change.

MJ: What were some of the foundational ideas and concepts that informed the creation of the "Courage to Teach" retreats that you brought forward into the retreat you developed for the physicians and medical educators who were ACGME awardees?

PJP: There are several things I could say about that but let me start with one of

Courage to Grow

David Leach, MD
Past Executive Director of the Accreditation Council for Graduate Medical
Education

Good things get better as you get closer to them; bad things get worse. My first encounter with Parker Palmer was via a DVD of a speech he had given at the Institute for Healthcare Improvement and from reading his books, my second was a phone conversation, and my third was a personal encounter when he facilitated a retreat for residency program directors. Each encounter brought me closer to him and I knew that not only was he good but also that he would have a major impact on my life.

If I were a tree I would have noticed that my roots were being nourished. Most things in academic medicine stimulate "foliage" (performance indicators, publications, grants, titles, promotions, etc.); "roots" (values, deeply held truths and beliefs, altruism, professionalism, etc.) are assumed but are usually not attended to with as much care. Parker was attentive to my roots and taught me the power of "living divided no more." He clarified for me that my frustrations and my desire to improve things were motivated by love; I loved my profession too much to let it fall to its most degraded state. He gave me the tools to help me have conversations with my "inner teacher" and he taught me how to help others have conversations with their inner teacher. I learned about the courage that comes from clarity in community, especially a community living divided no more.

As a result I began to use poetry in my speeches and writings, I began to talk openly about values, and I began to think about resident education as formation, as a shaping experience that requires deep attention to both internal and external contexts. Life became much more interesting. I found that there was a tremendous hunger for conversations like this within the profession. A few years later I was given the Association of American Medical Colleges' Flexner Award, a form of foliage that depends on good roots. Thanks, Parker.

the ideas that has animated my work and our retreats: the power and importance of each of us living, to the extent possible, an undivided life. We live in a world where it feels threatening to let our own identity and integrity reveal itself. So we build this wall, partly for interior reasons, and then I think as we grow older we work our way through a series of institutions, especially schools and the workplace, where we are actively taught to keep that wall high and wide and thick. I think of all these folk sayings we have in our culture – "Don't wear your heart on your sleeve" or "Play your cards close to your vest" – that are all about how risky it is, how unsafe it is, to let your true identity be known in the world. The problem with this, obviously, is that the self (not the little ego self, the little selfish self, but the true self, the self as we were meant to be) wants to make itself known in the world because ultimately it's the only gift we have to give.

Primacy of True Self

Hanna Sherman, MD
Program Director, Health Care Programs, Center for Courage and Renewal

At the end of 1999 I was at a transition point in my career. As I considered how I wanted to shape the next phase of my work, I wanted to eliminate the compartmentalization I felt in my professional and personal lives. I didn't realize what I was seeking was to live undivided until I began reading Parker's work and recognized in his words how I felt. At the same time, I became concerned about physician burnout and well-being and the care we were giving our patients. With many of my friends and colleagues feeling beleaguered and disaffected from medicine, how could we be the healers and role models that our patients needed us to be?

A medical student once told me that she was considering leaving school because she felt she was losing pieces of herself. I vowed at that time to do what I could to prevent that loss of self, for myself and for other physicians.

I really believe that the gift we have to give to each other and to the world is not first and foremost in the skills that we went to school to learn, the trained capacities that we've developed. Those are valuable, sure enough, but the selfhood that we can offer each other, the gift of identity and integrity, the gift of presence, is one way that a lot of the wisdom traditions have put it – that's what we have to offer. And to live a life in which you're not offering that gift, I think, falls short of why we are here, who we were meant to be and how we were meant to be.

We also know that in the important work that people do in the world, the gift of self isn't just about the self-satisfaction of the person giving the gift. It's about the goodness of the work itself. We know for a fact that a doctor who brings herself or himself into the relationship with a patient is a more effective healer than a doctor who only brings in information and technique. Because then the patient ends up feeling like an object rather than a person, and the patient's full powers of personhood are not invoked and evoked for healing – the spiritual and psychological and mental powers that we know from clinical research are such an important part of the healing equation. Only a doctor who is fully present as herself or himself in a relationship can evoke that.

MJ: Does this individual transformation link in any way to institutional formation? If so, how would you describe your theory of change?

PJP: Our theory of change certainly begins with that work of individual transformation, which we don't force on people; people have to choose that. People have to enter a free and safe space to let that emerge within themselves. That's what formation in a Circle of Trust is all about. But the Circle of Trust is also about a community of folks who both evoke that inner work from each other and then support and affirm each other, bless each other really, in carrying that inner work forward in institutional settings.

I believe that the work we help people do inwardly has consequences in the larger world. I not only believe that, I've seen it happen, in the lives of teachers, in the lives of physicians, in the lives of clergy who go back to their institutions not only with personally renewed hearts, but also with new ways of being in the world that spread renewal to others, which create community, and it is out of the ferment I think of that community that real change comes. If I hadn't seen that with my own eyes, I just would have had to find some honest way to make a living.

The title of my book *A Hidden Wholeness*[2] comes originally from a quote by Thomas Merton, who basically said, "In the midst of all the brokenness of the world, there is a hidden wholeness beneath the surface." It's easy to fall into despair if you care about what's going on in the world or in education or in religious institutions or in medical practice or any of these particular places that people care about. But Merton's affirmation is that somehow underneath the broken appearance of things, there is a wholeness that is hidden but is still there to be recovered, to be reclaimed. And for me the starting point of that, always, is to be recovered and reclaimed within ourselves, within each individual self. It seems to me that there is no way to work toward the wholeness of communities, and of institutions, and of societies, without starting with the individuals who make those things up.

MJ: Tell me about your first experience working with physicians and medical educators who were ACGME awardees. What was similar and what was unique about this group compared with groups of educators you'd worked with before?

PJP: It's a fascinating question because I went into that retreat with a little fear and trembling, thinking that the physicians were sort of a different species from regular human beings – carrying, I think, the kind of attitude of the typical patient toward the physician, as if they're sort of godlike, and possess all kinds of esoteric knowledge that would make it difficult to talk with him or her. But as you know, one of the things that I don't do going into retreats is to read people's résumés, because my approach to retreat leadership is that I don't want to be looking at them through their credentials, or the schools they went to, or the awards they've won. I just want to be looking them in the eyes – seeing their souls more than their roles.

And basically, I came out of that retreat realizing that there were a lot of similarities between working with physicians and working with K-12 teachers. In fact, at the end of the retreat one of the physicians said to me, "I suppose this was very different from working with K-12 teachers." And I said, "Well, it really wasn't." Of course, there were some particular differences in the case study we used or the examples we put forward, but fundamentally this was the same retreat. And part of that goes back to the fact that when I started working with K-12 teachers, I wasn't a K-12 teacher, just as I will never be a physician. But I learned something with the K-12 teachers that helped me with the physicians, which is that I don't need to possess the knowledge that allows them to inhabit their roles. What I can offer them is a way of evoking soul, or identity, or integrity, or selfhood, or inwardness – whatever you want to call it, that is such an important component of every professional practice. It's the joining of soul and role, the joining of the skill and the knowledge on one hand, and the identity and integrity of the selfhood of the person on the other, that makes the practice holistic – whether it's a teaching practice or a medical practice.

One participant put it this way: Normally when we come together as colleagues we talk about programs, techniques, and resources but here we were able to explore our lives and work in a way that allowed me to reclaim my core sense of Self that animated me to choose *this* vocation.

MJ: You mentioned using a case study with this group. How did you approach that?

PJP: One of my most vivid memories from that retreat was putting a case study before them of the breakdown of a health care system. The case study was around a particular patient who died, who should not have died; the death was a matter of medical error and neglect. This case was prepared with the help of a couple of the physicians in the group so that we had all the facts straight and . . . they were available from the public record, because this case had been litigated.

And I remember saying, "Now, we're going to read through this. And as we do, I know what you're going to be thinking about it. You're going to be thinking about a systems analysis that you're so skilled at doing. You think this way all the time. And when we're finished with the case, you're going to want to talk about what caused the failure of the system. But that's not what I want you to talk about. What I want you to talk about, as you go through the case, is what caused the failure of the healer's heart? Because in this case it was a resident who was responsible, and her supervisors, and the other physicians who were in her orbit, who had heart failure – who failed to live up to their Hippocratic oath to do no harm and ended up doing a lot of harm. "So my question is going to be: What caused the failure of the healer's heart? What might have been done in anticipation of this moment during residency train-ing itself, the kinds of programs that you're all leading, to mitigate against that heart failure? What might have been done in the moment by the resident, the healer, who could see the wheels falling off around her, and who might have responded differently to the crisis? What might have been done *after* the event to assure to the greatest extent possible that this kind of failure of the healer's heart didn't happen again?"

But what I remember is they had a *very* difficult time getting focused on that second question – or making a shift from the first to the second. And I had to intervene several times, and say, "No. You're doing a systems analysis. That's too easy. I want you to do the heart failure analysis." We eventually had some real breakthroughs. And I think there were some who left the retreat still wrestling with what does that even mean? But I think there were many who got a new set of lenses that day, who realized, "Oh, we can look at a case like this from both angles, through both lenses."

And then you link that back to an educational process, which either works with the heart of the healer in some systematic formative ways or fails to do so in ways that have consequences down the road. Is there anything that can be done in education to increase the student's sensitivity to the plight of the patient? Is there anything that can be done in education to increase the stu-dent's outrage about the way systems fail individuals? Is there anything that can be done in education to increase the student's sense of agency and power over those moments when the system is failing?

I think the answer to all of those questions is yes.

This case made me think a lot about the fact that transformation in so many of our major institutions is going to have to come from the profession-als who are at the heart of those operations. It seems clear that change will only come when we educate professionals to be not only competent in their professional practice, as I am sure this resident was (and I am quite sure all would have been well if she'd had a manageable case load), but how do we educate professionals not only to be competent in their professions but also to have competency and concern about transforming the dysfunctional insti-tutional conditions that allow things like this to happen? That starts, I think, with raising holy hell.

When your professional standards are violated, when you know that the institution has put you into a position where you cannot honor your Hippocratic oath, or whatever the equivalent of that is in your line of work, it raises the question: How do we educate professionals who know how to engage in long-term institutional transformation – in the very institutions that are making the professions we care about struggle to live up to their highest standards?

MJ: What other methods did you use in the retreat?

PJP: One of the standard features of the retreats that we do in this work is something called a "Clearness Committee," and I always like to say to people, "It sounds like it comes straight out of the '60s" and it does, but it's the 1660s, not the 1960s. It's a 300- to 400-year-old Quaker practice in which five or six people gather for 2 hours with a person who's got a question that he or she is wrestling with – an issue, a problem, a decision or discernment they're trying to make. For 2 full hours those five or six caring, competent adults operate with a very simple rule: they cannot speak to the "focus person" (the person with the issue) in any other way except to ask honest, open questions.

It sounds simple, but if you imagine not only the length of time involved (2 hours), and what's involved in asking honest, open questions, it turns out to be very challenging and demanding. "Have you thought about seeing a therapist?" is not an honest, open question. It represents the kind of question we like to ask, which has built-in advice. We often frame something as a question when in fact we are trying to advise someone. And the purpose of this process is to lay all of our advice aside, all of our wisdom, all of our guidance, all of our thoughts about what this person ought to do, and to create a space that is to be occupied by that person, and that person alone – so he or she can listen as closely as possible to his or her inner teacher, aided by questions that strip away whatever obstacles may lie between his or her inward truth. It's an extraordinary experience.

I remember when I first started learning about the Clearness Committee. I was in an academic setting; I was a university professor. It came very powerfully to me that this was simply an inquiry model, that it mirrored exactly the way great scholars in every field approach their subjects. You don't become a great scholar by telling subatomic particles what they are, or by telling historical data what they mean. You become a great scholar by listening, by asking, by asking honest, open questions of those subatomic particles or of those historical data. Who are you? What do you have to say to me? What do you have to say about yourselves? How do you define yourselves? Great scholarship comes from that open, honest inquiry that's mirrored in the Clearness Committee.

I think every wisdom tradition and its practices can be demonstrated to be a mode of knowing of ourselves and of the world, that is easily transported from a so-called sacred to a so-called secular tradition. Because that distinction doesn't really exist when we understand that what these wisdom traditions are all about at bottom is not an ethic, a set of "how we ought to be," but deeper than that, a way of knowing reality that opens up for us this hidden wholeness that's in ourselves and in our world.

MJ: What do you see as the benefits of the Clearness Committee?

PJP: There is obvious huge benefit for the focus person, but what's so interesting is that there is great benefit for everyone who participates in that process. People constantly tell us, "By following this discipline of asking honest, open questions, of trying to be fully present to this person, by laying aside my own tendency to want to give advice and fix people up, I learn so much myself and I learn so much about how I might relate to other people. And in reaching for those questions I had to journey back into my own life, and found that somewhere all of our lives draw on the same aquifer. As different as they may appear to be on the surface, we're all struggling with such similar things at bottom, at root." So, the Clearness Committee is in a lot of ways a microcosm of the whole Circle of Trust process [described later in the interview]. And when we ask people, as we've been doing for more than a decade now, "Of all the things we did in a Circle of Trust, the working with poetry, the silence, the journaling, the small groups, what would you say is the pearl of great price?" so many people say it was the Clearness Committee that brought this all home and that really was transformative. And at the heart of that Clearness Committee process is this very demanding discipline of asking honest, open questions.

MJ: When we prepare groups for Clearness Committees we help people learn the skill of asking honest, open questions – questions that have no agenda or disguised advice but which are intended to draw out the wisdom of the other person. What is an honest, open question or two that you'd like to ask of medical educators or health care professionals?

PJP: Given what I've just said, and if I begin with the assumption (which I believe to be true) that a lot of deeply thoughtful health care professionals are in a state of discouragement these days – caught in a contradiction between the kind of medicine they value and want to practice and the kind that is being forced upon them by institutional realities, private and public – I think the kind of honest, open question I would want to ask would be related to "How do you handle your heartbreak?"

And that leads to a series of other honest, open questions related to heartbreak: Is it turning you into a cynic? Is it hardening your heart? How well do you like yourself as a doctor? And what are those feelings all about? What resources are within your reach to help you hold the heartbreak in a more generative and creative way? Or if you're holding it in a creative way, what would you like to see other people have access to that has been helpful to you?

And the responses could be anything from that support group to the penalty-free zone for reporting medical errors that some health systems now have. But it seems to me that in every case I know of there's an intimate relationship between that support group of colleagues and the establishment of an institutional penalty-free zone, to take that example, because institutions don't do that of their own accord. They do it because courageous change agents within an organization say, "We've got to have this."

I'm sure there are a thousand honest, open questions that I would want to ask in a thousand different situations but that is where I'd start: "How are you handling your heartbreak?" Because as you know, for me, there are two ways for the heart to break. It can break open to greater capacity or break apart into a thousand pieces. And in some ways I think our retreats draw people who feel like they're on the edge of their heart breaking apart, and they want to learn to hold that experience in a way that helps it break open to greater capacity – to hold more of what they value and treasure about their work and the opportunities it provides. And the suffering that comes with it. To hold all of that in a life-giving way.

Clearness Committee Redux

Thomas S. Inui, ScM, MD

I was introduced to the tradition of Clearness Committees 13 years ago by Parker Palmer and colleagues at a Courage to Teach retreat conducted for the Fetzer Senior Scholars in Kalamazoo, Michigan. On this occasion, a remarkably diverse and talented group of individuals had gathered to share learning, grow as individuals, and become acquainted with various mindfulness practices. The Clearness Committee exercise Parker conducted with the Scholars was one I found instantly attractive. I had attended a Quaker men's college (Haverford College) where Meeting was mandatory and Clearness Committees were a part of the life of the culture. The Quaker educational philosophy of freedom, honor, and responsibility for community had deeply impressed me. The Clearness Committee, in its own way, was a "microcommunity" in which the asking of open and honest questions served the individual who had convened his or her trusted colleagues.

Lacking a suitable practice community, Quaker or otherwise, I have had no opportunity to pursue the formal Clearness Committee process since that exercise years ago. I have, however, adopted the "open and honest questioning" method for other activities of which I am regularly immersed. For example, I use this approach when mentoring faculty, graduate students, or undergraduate medical students. A mentor in my opinion should not imagine that he or she "knows everything" or even what might be best for the individual sitting before him or her. Instead, a mentor's experience may allow the mentor to broaden the mentee's vision of potential pathways lying ahead and to do his or her best to facilitate clearness on the part of the mentee about what is most important to the mentee.

I have also used "open and honest questioning" in facilitating student discussions in the professionalism seminars that are part of undergraduate medical education at the Indiana University School of Medicine. In these seminars, a small group of 12–14 students gather, have an opportunity to read one another's professionalism journal entries, and choose several entries to discuss as a group. My role in this process has been described elsewhere.[3] It is largely "open and honest questioning," including such questions as:

- What was it about this situation that attracted your attention?
- Why did this particular set of events unfold?
- Have any of the rest of you (student peers) seen something like this?
- What did it make you think at the time?
- How did you feel in the moment? Now?
- What were the choices in this situation?
- Would you make the same choices that you saw someone else make? If not, why not?
- In this situation what would you actually say if you wanted to change what was done?
- What are the risks of doing or saying something different? What are the risks of not doing something different?

As I recall Parker observing years ago, the most difficult aspect of the Clearness Committee process is to avoid asking questions that are "veiled suggestions." I remember this whenever the "doctor in me" wants to intervene in this seminar by suggesting a correct interpretation, the most appropriate action, or what would be best to think about a situation. Finding clearness with others involves minimizing one's own acts of ego in what I would be tempted to call "loving service."

MJ: Do any other interactions or experiences stand out from that first retreat with physicians?

PJP: One other thing that I will mention is we did have this closing circle of evaluations, values, and comments. What was this like for you? What did you like best? And there was one gentleman in the circle who had been silent through the retreat, and because I don't read people's résumés, I had no idea who he was. But in that closing circle, he spoke for the first time. And he said, "I went into medicine maybe 40 or 45 years ago, and the medicine I'm being asked to practice today, and the health care system I'm in, is a very different medicine than the one I signed up for. It's not why I came to this profession, and it's not what I value."

He went on to say, "I'm sixty-some years old and I don't know how much time and energy I have left, but it's very clear to me after this retreat that I want to spend my remaining time and energy trying to spread this sort of conversation and experience among more and more physicians. Because I think *this* is the kind of thing that can lead us out of the woods." And by that I think he meant both the processes that we had been using, which invited truth telling and shared exploration of important issues, and some of the ways of framing that exploration – like the heart failure versus the systems failure.

Later I asked David Leach who that was. And he gave me his name and then I asked, "What does he do?" "He's a heavyweight in a very important organization in American medicine," he said.

And here's one other story about this amazing man, which connects directly to the retreat and to his experience of the retreat. A few years later, when the ACGME reduced the duty hours for residents from 120 to 80, they were met with enormous resistance from health care institutions, residency programs, and the community.

There was a meeting in Chicago where this issue arose in open conversation with a good deal of heat and contentiousness, just before this man was to speak. So when he got up to speak, with the issues still hanging in the air, he said, "I'm going to throw away my prepared notes because I want to address what just happened here in the conversation you were just engaged in." And the gist of what he had to say was, "I will tell you what you need to do with the extra 40 hours a week you now have, with your work week reduced from 120 to 80. You need to learn to love," and he went on to say what that meant in a nonsentimental way.

I think that these retreats, starting from that very first one, really have been about a nonsentimental version of learning to love, in the midst of a medical practice, or in teaching – in the midst of teaching people who are headed for medical practice, learning to love in a way that has wheels on it, that isn't just exhortation, or fluff, or sentimentality, but is really about connecting with patients and families at very difficult moments and at very hard times, and bringing your full self along with your full knowledge and skill set to this very challenging practice of medicine.

MJ: As more interest developed in the health care sector we began preparing facilitators to lead Circles of Trust, primarily in health care. What are Circles of Trust?

PJP: Our approach to formation involves a group of people coming together in what we call "Circles of Trust." When I was writing the book *A Hidden Wholeness*[2] and I was searching for a name that would describe this form of community where we invite people "into being alone together" (where individuals can experience the solitude conducive to deep self-reflection within a supportive community of like-minded individuals), of making a space that honors the inner truth of every individual in the community, the phrase "Circle of Trust" came very quickly to mind. And while I think it's powerfully descriptive of what ultimately happens in these circles, I am also respectful of people who say, "Well, just because you call it a Circle of Trust doesn't mean that trust is going to happen," and in fact, trust at this level is very countercultural in our world. But what I think we do by calling it a "Circle of Trust" is precisely what Lincoln had in mind when he said, "We must invite the better angels of our nature onto the playing field," and into the public arena, opening our better self to others. I think like everything we do, this is invitational. It invites that trusting and trustworthy part of ourselves to show up.

MJ: Can you say something about how people relate to each other in a Circle of Trust?

PJP: We do follow some specific guidelines.

- *Clear Limits and Boundaries*: We try to be clear with people about how much time they are asked to give to this, and then we try to keep time very carefully. I think one of the things that makes the soul feel safe is leadership that comes through on its promises, and one of the promises we make is how we're going to use that time.
- *Intentionality*: There's another piece that has to do with the intentionality of this group, of why we're together. And clarity about the ground rules is what makes all of that possible.
- *Open Invitations*: A Circle of Trust must be invitational, openly invitational. This is not something that an employer can assign employees to do, and once people get there, everything that we do with them is offered up as an invitation where they have freedom of choice. This is not a "share or die" proposition!
- *No Fixing*: People in our society are constantly trying to fix each other, or save each other, or correct each other, or give advice. *Not* doing this is one of the hardest things for those of us in the "helping professions," but it is vital to welcoming the soul, to making space for the inner teacher.
- *Common Ground*: Seasonal metaphors have provided common ground and a way of framing the inner-life journey. Whatever our ideological, philosophical or religious differences may be, we are all embedded as human beings in the cycles of the seasons, and that gives us a way to talk about inner life issues in a pluralistic society.

- *Skilled Leadership*: Facilitation of these circles is very demanding because in many ways you're trying to hold back the tide: the tide of an awful lot of Western problem solving, invasive and evasive culture – invasive when we think we can fix something, and evasive when we realize we can't. It's one of the most demanding forms of leadership that I've ever attempted in my life.

More than this, I think one of the great wounds in our society is people feeling that they are treated as a means to some other end and never as an end in themselves. And I think it is incredibly wounding to be treated that way all your life. It's been moving to those of us who have done this work to hear teachers and doctors and lawyers and others say at the end of this journey we take together: "This is the first time in my life I haven't felt like a problem to be fixed, but rather a person to be honored."

The relationships in a Circle of Trust, it seems to me, can be likened, in kind of a startling way, to the experience many people have had sitting at the bedside of a dying person. I've talked with a lot of folks who've had that experience, and I've had that experience myself. In that ultimate moment with a dying person we discover two things that are very important, and that can carry over into other aspects of our lives. We first of all discover that we have to give up all of our problem-solving habits in order to be there in a helpful way, because this isn't a problem that we can solve. We don't have a fix for this one, the way we think we do for other problems that people have. And so I have asked a lot of people, "OK, you're not there trying to fix a problem that you can't fix. How are you there? In what manner are you there?" And the only word I have ever heard people use is the word "presence": "I was simply attempting to be present. I was trying to be fully present. I was trying to bring the whole of myself to this situation, this relationship, this moment in life."

When people learn these things, sitting at the bedside of a dying person or sitting in a Circle of Trust, they so often say, "What I've learned here I can take into other relationships of my life; I can learn to be less invasive of my children and less evasive, either imagining that I can live their lives for them and straighten them out, or pretend that what's happening isn't happening. I can learn to practice presence with my children, with my friends, with my spouse, with my colleagues, with anyone I meet." And when I think about those deathbed moments, I often think to myself: Why wait until the last few hours to practice this healthy way of being together, this respectful way of being together, paradoxically, this life-giving way of being together? Why wait for the last few hours? Why not start doing it right now?

Courage to be Vulnerable Together

Hanna Sherman, MD

In working with a wide range of health care professionals, I have seen individuals and teams improve their working relationships after learning to be in a Circle of Trust together. By sharing of their own identities and asking each other honest, open questions about issues of importance to them, the level of trust that ensues is profound and unlike anything they have experienced, especially in a hospital or practice environment. I think part of the transformation that has particular significance is the ability to be vulnerable together, to be honest about the risks and challenges of caring for patients and making difficult decisions for health care delivery.

MJ: You've written about the importance of developing greater capacity to hold the tensions in our lives – including our own suffering – as an alternative to violence. How is this capacity supported by Circles of Trust?

PJP: I think it's pretty obvious to a lot of people that we live in very broken times. We live in times with lots and lots of gaps between the difficult realities of life and what we know to be possible humanly. We know that we live in a world at war; we also know that it is possible to live at peace. That's a big example. We know that we live in a situation where health care is not as available to the people who need it most, and we know that humanly it would be possible to make it available. On and on and on it goes. Everybody would have their own example of what I've come to call these "tragic gaps." And I've come to believe that one of the most important capacities that a person can have in our time is the capacity to stand in the tragic gap, however that may be defined in their lives – whether that person wants to take on leadership (whether that's positional leadership or non-positional leadership) or simply wants to help make this a better world. To stand between the hard reality of what's going on in my school, in the lives of my students, in my hospital, in the community that my religious organization serves, whatever it may be, and what we know is really possible because we've seen it from time to time – and to stand there without flipping out on either side, is to stand and act in the tragic gap.

So the capacity to stand in this tragic gap and to hold those tensions is to me one of the great human qualities that I think we help cultivate in Circles of Trust. By giving people more access to that inner ground where you can stand and hold what appear to be radical opposites, we help them become a co-creative agent of finding a new way through, a new way ahead.

MJ: Let's talk about the kinds of challenges or concerns that arose from working with physicians and others in health care.

PJP: Well, I think one of the things it brings up which you and I have talked about often, and I've heard others talk about, is the challenge that some of the physician facilitators find in knowing what kind of language to put to this work that will communicate well with their colleagues. And as you know, this is a question to which I bring my own biases. Because, probably 30 years ago, before there was a Center for Courage & Renewal, or before there was Courage to Teach, I was talking about spirituality in higher education – which was not at the time a popular topic. It's now become a very popular topic, with all kinds of high-profile people aligning themselves with it. But I was simply feeling the need to name in a variety of ways what . . . what I sometimes called "the depth dimension" of higher education. To say that the complexities of modern life and the challenges faced by our students were just too deep to tolerate a higher education that stayed on the surface of things, with just the facts and the figures and the theoretical apparatus that helps you deal with all that. As it were, just the science of it. That we needed to go also to the humanistic side of things, the dimensions of heart and soul. The dimensions of selfhood that allow and encourage, let's say, an engineering student to go out into the world and not build shabby bridges that are going to collapse 10 years down the road. Or an accountancy student to go out into the world and refuse to cook the books for Enron. I think there are all kinds of critical professional issues at stake in the kind of education we give preprofessional people. And when you talk about them in the early days of a movement, of really a reform movement, people think you're nuts.

And you need to work hard to talk about them in ways that slip beneath the radar. So instead of talking about spirituality in higher education, I would talk about epistemology, about ways of knowing. Because I found that that language didn't make academics resistant, or make them scoff. That language would allow me to go to many of the same places that I wanted to go in terms of spirituality.

So I appreciate the dilemma that some of our physician-facilitators have in putting language to it. But at the same time, I think there is some language in the profession already that works with a lot of people. One such word is *professionalism*. I don't see the ACGME or anybody else having trouble using the notion of professionalism, which is, in effect, this dimension of depth that I talked about earlier. It means more than just the science. It means also the relation of dimensions and the selfhood and the heart and soul, the feeling.

Seeing Myself as a Creative Person

Val Ulstad, MD, MPH, MPA
Chief Engagement Officer, Partners at Cascade Bluff

When I first started to be involved with this work I had almost an allergic reaction to poetry. It represented something I didn't understand and something I assumed probably everyone else did. This, of course, triggered a favorite feeling (hear the sarcasm) of mine and of physicians in general: incompetence! Now in virtually everything I do, I use poetry, metaphors and stories to invite people to learn what they already know deeply – which is what Courage work did for me. Courage work has helped me get clearer about my professional calling as a physician educator and has helped me stay true in disorienting times. Deep personal reflective work with the resources of others in community has also helped me see myself as a creative person (not something my medical training did). This has helped me shape my personal and professional contributions over the course of the last 10 years into (for me) a deeply coherent and joyful life that feels (as Parker would say) "divided no more." Two years ago, after more than 20 years as a clinical cardiologist in academic and private practice settings, I shifted to another form of heart practice. Now my profession is relational and contextual work with individuals, groups, and organizations, hopefully helping others develop clarity of purpose, build their capacity to hold the tension of paradox, and increase their willingness to embrace a sense of possibility. I now call myself an educator in independent practice – an idea I got from Judy Brown, an elder mentor in Courage work. Through this work I have created a life that honors my passion for facilitating learning and for building my own and the capacity in others to be resilient and resourceful in the face of uncertainty and ambiguity.

MJ: You've been speaking about the importance of finding language that bridges – language that doesn't leave out the scientific mind but which is also able to bring in the other side, which is the heart and spirit of medicine. What else can you say about that?

PJP: Well, I think transformational work of this sort simply calls for pioneers who are willing to take risks. We need the Lewis and Clarks. People who are willing to say, "There's something out there. Don't know what it is. Don't know how to get to it, but we're going to walk into the wilderness." And others may stay behind and say, "They're nuts, they don't know what they're talking about. We're not going to follow them." But then they discover things.

And I think our use of language is something like that. So one of the things that I've seen, looking back on 30 or 40 years of working on spirituality in higher education, is that way back when – when that was a topic that kind of got laughed out of town – there were thousands of people *wanting* to talk that way, but not knowing they could, or not knowing how to do it. So language has to lead some of the time; it doesn't always follow where people are. It sometimes leads – into places that people then want to move toward.

Another thing I would say is the fact that there are – as far as I can tell – highly functional synonyms for some of the things we're trying to talk about. "Relationship-Centered health care" seems to have quite a following in medicine; "humanistic medical practice" seems to be in common usage; "professionalism," as we noted earlier. And it's my understanding that we have clinical evidence that physicians who relate with patients as whole persons get better results than physicians who simply treat patients as machines to be fixed.

MJ: Physicians are trained to be healers, and yet they often find themselves with patients or in situations where the kind of healing they would wish to bring about simply isn't possible. That has to be heartbreaking. You've written a lot about heartbreak and also about the many ways our heart can be broken open into greater capaciousness and compassion. How might that apply here?

PJP: In education we need so badly to learn to hold together this paradox between the mind and the heart, between the analytic mind and the feelingful heart. We need faculties in medical schools who can model a heartful response to profound life moments that a physician witnesses and intervenes in, perhaps every day of his or her life. Moments so profound, with such frequency that most of us – myself included – can't imagine what that would be like.

Unfortunately, we know what happens in professions where that's the constant experience. And what happens is people develop a very tough shell; they put on a thick mask. They shut down the feeling function. And I think I'm not wrong in saying that medicine has an abysmal record when it comes to alcohol and drug abuse among practitioners. Well, that's part of their self-anesthetizing that comes from not knowing how to hold these profoundly challenging emotional moments. My bet is that if you did a cost-benefit analysis of what it costs us to treat lots and lots of health care folks in poor health themselves – because they eat too much, or smoke too much, or drink too much, or they do too many drugs – to cover over the symptoms of having to deal with a lot of grief every day, it would be much less costly to have educational programs that not only prepare people better, but that also help them learn how to put together their own support systems. And if we could help health care systems learn how important support systems might be, it would more than pay for itself. I mean, why don't we have grief groups for doctors, as well as for the parents of children with certain illnesses, or the spouses of folks who have recently died? I think the cost-benefit analysis would really come out on the side of it being more economical to prepare for these things and teach health care professionals some ongoing tools about how to work with these things.

MJ: In the Tenth Anniversary Edition of *The Courage to Teach*,[1] and also in *Change* magazine, from the Carnegie Foundation for the Advancement of Teaching and Learning, you wrote about "the new professional."[4] How does that relate to medicine?

PJP: Yes, I make the case that no matter what profession you're looking at, the highest values of all of our professions are most threatened by the institutions that house those professions – that the threat doesn't come from the outside. So if you're a lawyer, and you really got into this business because you want to pursue justice, you're constantly finding yourself thwarted by the legal system, which turns it into a chess game rather than a pursuit of justice. If you're a teacher who wants to serve kids, you're thwarted by a school system which values high-stakes testing more than dealing with individual student needs. And if you're a physician, you're thwarted by a health care system that does all of the things we've been talking about here that get in the way of . . . well, ultimately, of the Hippocratic oath.

I argue that it's no longer enough for professional education to focus exclusively on the core knowledge and skills necessary to practice the profession. Professional education must also focus on some of the rudimentary skills and sensibilities it takes to become a change agent within institutions.

I think some of it has to do with emotional intelligence. And getting in touch with our true feelings may help us see that some of our most precious professional values are distorted by the system in which we are working. It's also important to develop those kinds of relational skills that allow us to band together because change doesn't come from one person's conscience or one person's good will.

And I would loop this back to our groups, to formation work and Circles of Trust, by saying that I think many of the things I call for in the article about the "new professional" are actually modeled and practiced in Circles of Trust. So there's a significant way in which our work provides the kind of experimental "farm" in which to develop the skills and sensibilities necessary to become a change agent within institutions. You open up the feeling side of you, you open up the relational side. You learn something about the power of the group to pursue a goal that individuals can't pursue as readily alone. So I think there's a nice connection there in terms of the transformation of medical education.

References

1. Palmer PJ. *The Courage to Teach: Exploring the Inner Landscape of a Teacher's Life*. Tenth Anniversary ed. San Francisco, CA: Jossey-Bass; 2007.
2. Palmer PJ. *A Hidden Wholeness: The Journey Toward an Undivided Life*. San Francisco, CA: Jossey-Bass; 2004.
3. Inui TS, Cottingham AH, Frankel RM, *et al.* Supporting teaching and learning of professionalism: changing the educational environment and students' "navigational skills." In: Creuss RL, Creuss SR, Steinert Y, editors. *Teaching Medical Professionalism*. Cambridge: Cambridge University Press; 2009. pp. 108–23.
4. Palmer PJ. A new professional: the aims of education revisited. *Change*. 2007; **39**(6): 6–13.

2

From Freedom to Learn to Freedom to Innovate

The Harvard Macy Institute Story

Elizabeth G. Armstrong with Sylvia Barsion

Introduction

All around us we are told that our future rests with creating innovations to advance our economy, our nations, our schools, and our health care systems. The question most of us struggle with is, "Can we create innovators, and if so, how?" Clayton Christensen and his colleagues have taken care of the "nature" versus "nurture" conundrum, at least as far as an "innovator's DNA" is concerned, in their newest book.[1] There are indeed individuals who seem to be born with such "change agent DNA," but there are many more who, consciously or otherwise, have learned the key behaviors that lead to innovation. I believe I am fortunate enough to belong to the latter group and I happily serve as catalyst for others so they can follow their paths and passions.

This chapter begins with a description of the fortuitous path that opened my mind to new ways of thinking about education and ultimately led to the formation of the Harvard Macy Institute.[2,3] This is followed by a discussion of the key elements of course structure, pedagogy, small group work, and other elements that led to the creation of a community of like-minded, activist scholars (well before Facebook!).

Birth of the Harvard Macy Institute

Core Principles

My PhD dissertation focused on creating courses for science teachers in training that would foster their self-direction and their inner control over what and how they taught. Typically, young teachers were given science syllabi (some were called teacher-proof) that had to be followed without question, which created a classroom environment that stifled the very curiosity we were keen to create. After all, I was saying out loud to myself as I began to develop my doctoral research, "How could they teach inquiry-based learning behaviors without exhibiting them?" Carl Rogers' work *Freedom to Learn*[4] and that of other researchers looking at shifting locus of control from other-directed to self-directed learning were also highly influential as I shaped my graduate research goals and plan.

The educational event during my graduate studies that offered me a new way to think about adult learners occurred by chance when I accompanied my husband to a course at the Harvard Business School (HBS) one evening in 1971. As a graduate student he was invited to bring a spouse or "significant other" to an evening case study discussion. All visitors were asked to read a 20-page case on marketing prior to attending this class, as was the tradition in all MBA classes.

That class was the most exciting teaching and learning experience that I had ever had. I realized that using case studies forced student learning to be interactive and learner focused rather than teacher centered. The teacher was an orchestra leader of the discussion and as such, the students created the music and sometimes even rewrote the score. The teacher made sure all the perspectives surrounding the case could be heard. Within a real-life context, what was learned through case studies became clearly applicable beyond the classroom.

I soon inquired about the HBS's Executive Management program because I was considering whether to enroll in this program. Impressive to me was the fact that their programs included people from across the world and from different disciplines, and the faculty actively worked to keep participants forever connected. In fact, executive courses at the HBS were a far better pedagogical model than almost all of the graduate education courses I had experienced. My strong belief in experiential learning started at an early age, and I still feel that the best way for children and adults to learn is by actively engaging in their own learning processes. When students of any age appear to be unwilling participants in an "educational" program it is usually because the excitement of discovery, collaboration and reflection are not part of the experience. Why was I always seeing half empty lecture halls in graduate and medical schools around the country?

It became apparent to me through my observations, now ranging from elementary through graduate school, that teachers often *spoke* about their interest in creating self-directed and independent students; yet, there was little in their teaching that *demonstrated* that the teachers were self-directed, or that their teaching strategies nurtured that behavior. Teachers' were too likely to adhere to a prescribed syllabus regardless of student readiness or rely on an overly prescribed and didactic lecture format (devoid of hands-on experiences) when students were in need of more time to interact with each other, with the material and with their teachers.

My first medical school appointment was at the State University of New York at Stony Brook in the School of Allied Health Professions and in the School of Medicine. Five years later, when I accepted a position, first as an educator consultant, and then later as director of curriculum development at Harvard Medical School (HMS), I brought my enthusiasm for the case study method with me. In 1994 (after 10 years at HMS), I was appointed director of medical education at HMS. As my career progressed, I saw the same problems in the way continuing professional development (CPD) was conducted as I had observed in high school and college teaching. I was concerned by the routine workshops on "how to make effective slides" or "better ways to give feedback" that offered one method or template and encouraged very bright faculty to follow five to seven easy steps. Those workshops felt antithetical to creating innovators and self-directed educators. In addition, these programs were geared toward individuals who attended as solo educators. I believed that not only were such workshops limited, with respect to their lasting potential or meaningful impact for individuals, but also rarely were institutions or practices in the field affected by them after their studies. If faculty development programs were to have staying power then participants' organizations had to be influenced as well. I became increasingly convinced that even if faculty development programs were structured to make an important and lasting impact on individuals, there had to be an additional strategy specifically targeted to changing the organization.

The Macy Foundation Proposal

Daniel Tosteson, the dean of HMS from 1977 to 1997, launched an innovative New Pathway curriculum in 1985. It was, especially for that time, an enormous and innovative restructuring of medical education. Part of Tosteson's rationale for the New Pathway was his belief that medical students would learn better if they were responsible for their own learning rather than learning largely through lectures and texts. A primary vehicle to change the way students learned was the use of case studies and problem-based learning.

Dean Tosteson was keen to have this New Pathway create a revolution in medical education worldwide. Critical to the success of Harvard's New Pathway curriculum, for which a distinguished group of medical educators were originally hired, was the education of large numbers of faculty in new teaching methods. This challenge was made more interesting by the fact that faculty would need to understand why they were being asked to forego lecturing in favor of methods of case teaching that would require far more trust in the students' ability to be self-directed learners. This would require a significant shift in faculty attitudes and beliefs about how one learns. It was within this context that I was asked to write a grant proposal for funds to support professional development of faculty in a way that was consistent with the goals of the New Pathway. Specifically, I was asked to design a proposal to the Josiah Macy Jr. Foundation that would convey the excitement felt at HMS about the New Pathway and would make clear why the Foundation should fund the enormous educational revolution that we wanted to create. This was the chance of a lifetime and I said "yes," but I had no idea what those three little letters strung together in the right order would lead to.

In preparing myself to write the grant proposal, I reflected on the trajectory of medical education and the flaws I perceived in faculty preparation for teaching. We had a remarkable opportunity to not only disseminate ideas from the New Pathway but also to encourage faculty at other medical schools to innovate and create their own New Pathways – curricula that would work in their culture. From my perspective, the proposal should not be about helping everyone to model and adopt the New Pathway approach but rather to give others the skills, courage and impetus to be innovators and create perhaps even stronger models for their context.

The grant spelled out the creation of the Harvard Macy Institute (HMI). The goal was to create medical educators who were better problem-solvers, who could invent new solutions for their own institutions and take risks. The proposal included brief descriptions of two courses that became the backbone of the current HMI. One course was the Program for Physician Educators – geared toward on-the-ground teachers in medical education. In order to support educators and get approvals for new work at their home institution the leaders of those organizations also would have to be influenced. Hence, the Program for Leaders in Medical Education was proposed. We needed to have an effect on multiple layers of our organizations to have substantial change.

There were two other components of the original proposal. There was a Fellowship Program in Medical Education Reform, which offered individualized consultative support to a small number of senior leaders of major medical education reform efforts. The other component was support to teams of faculty from three to four institutions to work together on focused activities for a 1-week small symposium on topics such as ambulatory care education or patient-doctor courses. We recognized that most successful and lasting reforms are accomplished by teams rather than by individuals acting alone. HMI admissions policies and programs were designed to encourage participation by more than one person from the same institution, whether in the same or subsequent years.

Partners from Harvard Graduate School of Education and Harvard Business School

A member of the Foundation Board of Directors was a former dean of the Harvard Graduate School of Education (HGSE). She encouraged us to work with HGSE so that relationship could become an integral part of the grant proposal. At that time, Robert Kegan was the only faculty member studying adult development at HGSE. We could not have asked for a more brilliant and committed partner. He has been an essential part of the Educator course since that time. That course also quickly became the Program for Educators in the Health Professions, as we wanted to attract teams of health care professionals from multiple disciplines to attend – and they have.

Part of the design of the Leaders course involved attracting someone from the HBS to teach in the course. Not everyone at HMS at the time thought this was a great idea, but I did and I persevered. The challenge for me was to find the right person on the faculty who would be willing to come across the intellectual bridge from HBS to HMS. This was before the time that it was commonplace for medical schools to be collaborating with business schools even on the same university campus. Fortunately for us, Clayton Christensen had been introduced to me because of his disruptive innovation theory of organizational change[5] – this was before his first book came out. In fact, he was a very new HBS faculty member, having just finished his doctoral work. I called to make an appointment with him and the rest is history. The parallels between his work in industry and the problems I saw in both education and health care intrigued him. I know how important that first meeting was to both the HMI and me because he has led the leadership course with me ever since. It was only when I read the first page of his book *The Innovator's Prescription*[5] – where he talks about that original meeting with me – that I realized the impact on him. We are honored and privileged that Professor Christensen, whose work and books have won multiple international awards, continues to this day as a course director and a core member of the HMI team. He has also been influential in recruiting other leading expert faculty in health care change from HBS to our course. His passion for understanding and developing capacity for innovation is consistent with our mission, "creating a global community of health care educators and leaders dedicated to transforming health care delivery and education."

The Future in Four Pages

Drawing upon the collective power of the suggestions from a number of my "mentors" (this includes anyone who helped me question the status quo) and the distinguished team of medical educators at HMS, I submitted a four-page proposal that laid out the framework for the HMI. It represented my attempt to address the problem of the solo medical educator who needed a network and needed to be inspired to innovate if we were ever to create a revolution in education!

Toward a Self-Sustaining Model

Financing

The Macy Foundation approved the proposal and awarded us a grant in 1994 for $1.5 million over a 3-year period. After the first year, we realized we could not make the Institute self-sustaining, given the 12- to 18-month lead time needed to refine and market the programs or courses. We had just run the first set of courses. The costs were substantial. The first cohort of 25 physicians in the Educator program received a stipend and paid no tuition. We would need to continue to pay for faculty and for teaching space. It was clear that the initial business model for the courses was not going to work if we wanted the program to be self-sustaining.

I wrote to the Macy Foundation's new president, June Osborne, and told her that if she wanted this program to become institutionalized it needed additional support for a longer period than the original 3 years of funding.

It became clear that the program needed to lower net costs. That change was implemented right away. In the second year of the HMI, a stipend was not offered to those taking the courses. After that, the Institute started charging tuition. Dr. Osborne also asked me to write a second proposal. Because I believed we needed to continue innovating beyond the Boston-based courses, I thought we should create four regional centers, each with its own hub for an HMI-like program. The intent was to get others involved and create even more personal ownership of the HMI concepts. After all, we were all about building a community of scholar educators. That idea was wisely rejected by the Foundation because creating regional centers would stretch our limited HMI staff too thinly. We agreed that what was most needed was to concentrate on making the HMI a success in one location. The Macy Foundation was very generous in giving us support for 4 more years. They declared that was not their tradition – we broke new ground for them too. However, at this point they said that we would have to be on our own and self-sustaining when that second grant was over. Their support for the first 7 years paid off. The program has been self-sustaining since then – that is, from 2000 to the current day. And the wisdom of their investment is clear, given that the HMI program has influenced thousands of health care providers and educators along with hundreds of health care institutions worldwide.

The Macy Foundation grants provided an opportunity to create an ideal CPD program. It built on all of the founder's and the planning team members' experiences in education. I knew our team, comprised of educators, physicians, and professors from multiple professional schools at Harvard and around the country, could build a professional development opportunity that was different than anything available at the time. Our pedagogy, centered on experiential learning and enhanced by community and network building, provided opportunities for individuals and organizations to be transformed.

Course Structure

We created a unique structure for the Educators course, one that required translating theories into practice. Those applying to participate in an HMI course had to complete an application that required a description of an educational project approved at his or her home institution. The course began with a 10-day highly intensive learning experience, followed by 5 months back at one's home institution to work on the institutional project and apply what was learned, and then another 5 days of course sessions back at HMS with the same participants. There was nothing like this in 1995 when the first courses were offered and this structure is rare to this very day.

Becoming a Better Teacher

Robert A. Weber, MD
Professor and Vice-Chair of Education, Department of Surgery
Chief, Section of Hand Surgery
Scott & White Hospital, Texas A&M Health Science Center

I wasn't totally forthcoming. I told my dean that my goal was to design a faculty development program for our Department of Surgery, but I had an ulterior motive: to learn to be a better teacher. I was a residency program director, associate professor at the medical school, and busy surgeon. In short, like all of my colleagues, I was an active clinician who was expected to have a significant educational impact at our institution. I had done a great deal of teaching, enjoyed it, and had received feedback that I was good at it, but I had never been taught how to teach or received any formal education in adult learning.

Our university did not have any classes or training to offer, but an associate suggested I look into the Harvard Macy program. I enrolled in the Program for Educators in the Health Professions in 2006 expecting to pick up techniques to use in lectures, the operating room, and small group discussions. We learned that and much more. While principles and specific applications of adult education theory were the foundation of the program, the Institute taught us the fundamentals and importance of curriculum, assessment, and organizational change. My initial skepticism as to the

---

usefulness of such information changed when I saw how an understanding of these concepts placed my teaching in a context and opened new areas of education to explore. I learned how to Teach.

The time spent at the Harvard Macy Institute has had a significant impact on me, my institution, and my specialty. Five years after the course, I'm in a position not only to teach surgery but also to teach others how to teach. I believe I'm much better equipped to serve as the vice-chair of education and to be on the Accreditation Council for Graduate Medical Education Residency Review Committee for plastic surgery; the Department of Surgery has implemented the faculty development program I developed for my project at the Harvard Macy Institute, and the dean has asked to implement it for the entire institution (taught with another Harvard Macy scholar at our institution); and our specialty journal is in the process of publishing a series of articles on education in order to provide surgical colleagues the tools to be better teachers. Most important, the students say I'm a better teacher.

There's an old saying that goes, "Give a man a fish, and you feed him for a day. Teach a man how to fish, and you feed him for a lifetime." I'd add, "Teach a man how to teach others to fish, and you feed a whole village now and for generations to come."

The 5-and-a-half-day Leaders course employed the same pedagogical strategies as the Educators course but with a stronger focus on case studies and theory from business. A program, entitled A Systems Approach to Assessment in the Health Professions, a third HMI offering, was launched in 2007 with Constance Bowe, Louis Pangaro, and Thomas Aretz as codirectors with me. It is also a 5-and-a-half-day course. Participants are required to bring a significant assessment challenge their institution is facing that will serve as their focus for a number of small-group sessions. According to one participant in two recent HMI courses, "[HMI was] personally transformational, in that I am told I now both teach and assess in much better ways. These two programs are the best two time investments I have made in professional development, in my working life."

Pedagogy

We used pedagogical methods that had not previously been used in CPD programs. Each course requires deep immersion in the content and processes of personal and team learning experiences, with participants far removed from their daily lives. Sessions start early in the day and there is a full schedule until the evening, when assigned readings are to be done. For most, this is a rare opportunity to focus completely on what it means to be an educator in the health care professions. Stepping-back and reflection are taught, modeled, and encouraged.

Long-held assumptions about teaching, learning, and personal change are challenged.

Creating an Academy of Medical Educators: I Can Do That!

Darshana Shah, PhD
Associate Dean, Faculty Affairs and Professional Development Professor
Chief, Pathology Academic Section, Marshall University, Joan C. Edwards School of Medicine

As a course director in pathology, I saw faculty struggling to balance their teaching responsibilities with research and clinical service. Our medical school – a fairly young, state-funded school in the heart of Appalachia – did not have any programs supporting teachers. I had several ideas of ways to help my fellow teachers, but I hesitated to step forward with them; my perception was that my position was too low on the academic hierarchical ladder for me to recommend systemic changes. That was before my institution sent me to the Harvard Macy program for leaders in education in 2004.

Like every other participant, I came to the Harvard Macy Institute (HMI) with a project – more like an idea of what I would like to do for my fellow teachers. I hoped to get some tips and tools to get this project off the ground. Inspired by Dr. David Irby's work, I wanted to create an Academy of Medical Educators at my school, but the goal seemed out of reach: in 2004, there were only a handful of these academies, and they were at schools already blessed with power, prestige, and ample resources. The need to support teachers and make the "educational leg" visible was recognized, but other priorities always seemed to take precedence.

While interacting with HMI faculty and fellow scholars, I began to realize that in pursuing my dream of creating a platform for my fellow teachers, the biggest hindrance was not the location of the institution, my position, or the priority list: it was the boundaries I myself was drawing.

The first valuable lesson I learned at the HMI is that it is not where you sit on the hierarchical ladder that empowers you: wherever you are, empowerment comes from your ability to see beyond your position. The most surprising part is that you are transformed in the process without even realizing it. Suddenly every challenge looked like an opportunity to me. Terms like "lack of resources," "credential barriers," and "cultural barriers" were miraculously erased from my dictionary.

Case-based teaching with a business model of leadership is the unique aspect of the HMI course. It makes you think outside the box. Initially that may shake you out of your comfort zone, but eventually you begin to see similarities among many complex problems. Like other leadership courses, it is designed to teach several strategies to enhance your skill sets. However, the Harvard Macy course also taught me an additional lesson: always question your intentions, but never question your ability.

My HMI project of creating an academy of medical educators at Marshall became a reality just months after attending the HMI. Now in its eighth year with 48 members, our academy is a beacon that recognizes passionate teachers and promotes their growth. Certainly it has given great visibility to the "education leg" at the school. Our dean called its creation a landmark event that signified the importance of medical education in the mission of our medical school, and said academy members represent "the best among us" in their dedication to providing excellence in teaching.

Since the Academy's creation, its scope has grown: by incorporating faculty candidates from the university's College of Health Professions, it has added an important interdisciplinary dimension. As the university moves forward in creating a campus of health professions, the academy becomes a focal point for all educators.

Response from faculty has been quite positive. In fact, one compliment I particularly treasure applies perfectly to the HMI itself: "You will directly or indirectly leave behind a cadre of educators and educated students," wrote a retiring professor of medicine. "I am sure there will be a multiplier effect like a cascade of kinases."

As educators, we often do not model what we are preaching as the new way to learn and to teach. Thus, at HMI we carefully model in our small and large group sessions the strategies we want participants to learn. Facilitating highly interactive exchanges in a large group (now 75 scholars in many classes) at HMI demonstrates clearly how participants can do the same thing at their own institutions.

Multidisciplinary

Many at HMS did not see the need for collaboration with the HGSE and HBS, and at first many scholars did not want to read literature from "other" journals, especially the *Harvard Business Review*, which they argued was just for the business world. Those readings are now often the favorites in the courses. I am delighted that the courses took the risk of adding these collaborative features, because these readings and practices (such as the case study method learned at HBS) have become some of the strongest features of the HMI program. For example, it was working with Bob Kegan that led us to introduce faculty development that not only sought to attain the powerful goal of personal transformation for participants but also developed the unique structure and strategy to make that happen. And the collaboration with Clayton Christensen informs and inspires academic educators to apply the disruptive innovation theory to their work as teachers and clinicians.

Imagining What is Possible

Nelda S. Godfrey, PhD, RN, ACNS-BC
Associate Dean for Undergraduate Programs
Clinical Associate Professor
University of Kansas School of Nursing

As the associate dean of a large undergraduate nursing program, I found much of what we were teaching was fairly solid but that it was 'stale' in terms of a flow of new ideas. Introducing faculty to Collins' *Good To Great and the Social Sectors*[6] was like a breath of fresh air and it formed the framework for many faculty discussions. Presenting Kolb's learning theory in a more coherent way helped students and faculty have a better handle on the role of learning approaches in the educational enterprise. For us, the interface with the Schools of Business and Education presented at HMI directly affected our faculty's knowledge and ability to operate outside the provincialism of our own discipline.

However, the most dramatic example of innovation came, for us, in seeing what might be possible in terms of School of Medicine and School of Nursing collaboration. Academic societies had been in place in our School of Medicine for the past decade. In looking at their positive results, we started a professionalism initiative in the School of Nursing that included a rite of passage ceremony (not unlike the White Coat event in medicine) called the Nightingale Ceremony, and academic societies for School of Nursing undergraduates. Walking through Tosteson Hall and seeing the locations of the four societies at Harvard Medical School during the Harvard Macy Institute certainly made the idea of academic societies in nursing more real. However, without being able to *imagine* the collaboration between the School of Medicine and School of Nursing, none of this important educational work would be serving our students today.

I wanted the program to be interdisciplinary, knowing that the differing perspectives would enrich the course experiences for all. When we accepted a podiatrist as a participant, there were some who wondered about the need to have representatives from across the health care disciplines. Fortunately, not only was this podiatrist educator a wonderful participant and colleague but also he has become an innovator who created his pathway to becoming a successful dean. The case-based method of learning is still new for most of the participants, and it makes a strong impression.

Harvard Macy Institute Faculty

The notion of differing perspectives enriching the HMI program was exemplified most profoundly in the quality and diversity of the HMI course faculty. Tapping the talents of the faculty at other professional schools within the same university was seen as revolutionary in 1994. The proposal to the Macy Foundation said that in creating HMI, we should ask faculty whose professional goals aligned well with the mission of HMI, even if the faculty came from diverse fields within and outside of medical education. The diversity of talented faculty from multiple disciplines was a key to the HMI building its strong reputation for excellence and organizational change. While today most university presidents are advocating for more of this cross-pollination, they are still struggling with the university's rigid financial or organizational structures that prevent this synergy from happening.

Scholars

We called all the participants Scholars and we avoided using anyone's job title. This sent the message to participants that the readings, small group discussions, and overall level of discourse clearly were scholarly work. It also was a great equalizer: no matter what field within the health professions or the years of experience, all participants were seen equally as Scholars.

Faculty Alumni Scholars

A strategy created from the outset was to keep participants engaged in the work of the HMI by inviting them to return in future years as Faculty Alumni Scholars. In this role, they facilitate the critically important small group sessions, teach an elective which sometimes becomes a new element in the core of the curriculum, and are able to participate fully in the rest of the course. They have to pay for their own travel expenses, but in exchange for their significant contribution as faculty, they can experience the entire course again without the tuition cost. Faculty Alumni Scholars typically become more invested in the HMI and in the field of education for health care professionals. They are a great source of new ideas that keep the HMI innovative each year. They are key members of the community and we listen well to each other.

International Participation

Many at the medical school thought the HMI should be just for HMS faculty. I thought that would limit the kind of learning that had the potential of becoming transformational. Interestingly, Dean Tosteson wanted the New Pathway to revolutionize medical education on an international scale but the Macy Foundation felt its mission was more national. Over time, we convinced the Foundation that we would learn so much from what was going on elsewhere around the world.

Leadership for Innovation

Professor Steve Field, CBE, FRCP, FFPH, FRCGP
Chairman, NHS Future Forum
Chairman, National Health Inclusion Board
General practitioner, Bellevue Medical Centre Birmingham

I am proud to have been a delegate and, for the past 10 years, a member of the faculty for the Harvard Macy Institute (HMI) Leading Innovations in Health Care and Education programme.

My first contact with our course director, Dr. Elizabeth Armstrong, was as a delegate on a residential course in the United Kingdom for postgraduate medical deans and other medical educators delivered by the Association for the Study of Medical Education in partnership with the HMI. It was a tremendous success. Not only did we take tea and go to church with the Queen in Windsor but also we participated in a stimulating week of learning. It was one of the turning points in my career as a clinical educator and leader. I immediately signed up as a Scholar on the next leadership course run in Boston by HMI and that was another giant leap in my learning!

The HMI course worked on different levels. It introduced me to new teaching methods including the Harvard Case Method of teaching including cases from the nonmedical business world. It was on that course that I first met Clay Christensen of the Harvard Business School. That first course stretched my thinking and began my networking with fellow educators and clinical leaders from across the globe. It was a great honour, therefore, to be asked back the following year as a member of faculty. My annual visits have become the great intellectual highlight of each year.

The course develops organically year on year. It has been a privilege to work with Liz, Clay, and the other members of the faculty as the theory of 'Disruptive Innovation' has developed and had impact in and across the medical world. Ideas that were mainly confined to the business world have taken hold in the health systems of many countries. It has also been wonderful to see delegates go back to their home institutions and use the many ideas and techniques to reform their curricula and health care delivery systems.

I continue to learn new things and share ideas with the Harvard Macy community at conferences and across the net. I now have many close friendships with members of faculty and delegates that I regularly share thoughts with that have helped me with my career as a clinical leader.

For the 3 years that I led the world's biggest royal college (the Royal College of General Practitioners in the United Kingdom), the Harvard Macy community helped me with ideas for development of our training curriculum and in the development of policies for improving the quality of primary care in the United Kingdom.

On completing my term at the Royal College of General Practitioners, I was asked to lead the prime minister's review of the government's National Health Service (NHS) policy. The NHS Future Forum was launched on April 6, 2011, as part of the government's listening exercise on the Health and Social Care Bill. As its chairman, I led a 45-member team that in an 8-week period attended around 200 events and met more than 6700 people face to face. More than 25 000 people sent their views to the forum by e-mail, while a further 4000 sent private comments, completed questionnaires or website responses.

It was a highly sensitive and highly charged political commission in full view of the national media. I referred regularly to many of the papers that I have on file from the course and to Clay's books as I traveled England listening to patients and health care workers.

Writing and then finally delivering my final paper to the prime minister and the Cabinet at Downing Street was like writing and presenting a Harvard Case. Members of the Harvard Macy community commented on some of the drafts of the documents and lessons that I learnt while being a delegate and a member of faculty helped me with this ultimate task of advising our government on the future direction of the NHS in England.

Note: The final document, *NHS Future Forum: Summary Report on Proposed Changes to the NHS*, is available on the UK Department of Health website (www.dh.gov.uk/prod_consum_dh/groups/dh_digitalassets/documents/digitalasset/dh_127540.pdf)

Building Community

At the heart of the HMI was the desire to build a strong community of scholars who had a common interest in health care education and who would build a continuing and expanding base of expertise and innovation.

Related to creating a feeling of community is the need to recognize and respect the power of the team. Had the years put into creating and building on the HMI always been about "me" (remembering that I was asked to draft this chapter and forced to focus on me!), I am guessing the HMI would be a thing of the past. As it has happened, members of our HMI team get invited to places all over the world, are honored in the courses, are doing research, have been published[7-9] and have been promoted because of being part of this group of innovators. An innovation has to benefit all who are affected, especially those creating it, so there is a win-win-win situation for everyone, and honors for all.

Hopes

My hope when I wrote the proposal back in 1994 was to create a safe haven for the "black sheep" of academic research centers – the teachers! I wanted to build an international and interdisciplinary community that would take pride in its alumni network. I sought to increase the self-esteem of educators and in so doing their confidence and ability to foster change.

I wanted to advance a wide range of innovations (not a single template) in education across the whole continuum, advance innovations within the home institution, offer educators what I thought the scientists have – a network and new ways to collaborate across institutions and nations. I was heavily involved in "quality improvement" science and thought that those concepts should be brought to medical education as well. There is no reason to maintain the status quo when it is not working! I wanted all to benefit – the faculty and the scholars – and their institutions. I thought the HMI should become a learning experience for individuals and institutions.

When Reality Exceeds Expectations

Margaret Hay, PhD
Director, MBBS Admissions
Director, MBBS Assessment Data
Faculty of Medicine, Nursing and Health Sciences
Monash University Australia

It is a wonderful occurrence in life when a reality vastly exceeds one's expectations. Such is my experience with the Harvard Macy Institute (HMI). Although excited by the prospect of learning at Harvard University, I could never have envisaged all that has been instigated from my participation in the Harvard Macy community. I was an HMI Scholar in both the Educators and Assessment courses in 2010, and again in 2011 when I completed the Leaders course. I was also a returning Alumni Faculty member for the Educators and Assessment courses in 2011, both undertaken during my 6-month sabbatical at the HMI.

The rapid expansion at my institution from one medical school in 2002 with an annual intake of 140 to three medical schools (one international) and an annual intake presently around 500 provided the impetus for innovation and my interest in the HMI. The assessment processes designed for our original program were simply no longer feasible. Alternatives without loss of educational quality were required. I therefore came to the Harvard Macy courses with urgent and substantial educational challenges, and various amorphous ideas to meet them. These ideas were shaped into achievable realities through my HMI courses project group discussions, in concert with my immersion in the relevant and inspiring teachings that thread throughout these courses. The many in-depth discussions with fellow scholars from around the world further cemented these ideas.

I diligently applied the concepts learned during the HMI courses to successfully achieve a range of innovations in undergraduate medicine assessment at my institution. These innovations, born during the HMI Educators and Assessment courses, were designed to promote a sustainable effective teaching and learning environment within the preclinical years of my institution's medical degree initially, and have now extended to the clinical years. Taking a systems approach (learned during the HMI Assessment course), they were designed to coordinate with each other, through discipline leaders working together across our geographically dispersed model of curriculum implementation (including internationally). Such coordination was essential to the establishment of an effective learning environment within my institution's medical training program, and to the sustainability of the innovations through staff and student engagement. Specifically, these were the development of an innovative Objective Structured Clinical Examination for the preclinical years; the implementation of Google Apps (Education) as the secure platform for medical assessment item generation (using Google Docs), examiner and simulated patient standardization (using Google Video); electronic scoring via tablet computers; an entirely new system for management of assessment data; direct e-mail of individualized student performance feedback; and a substantial shift in the procedure for progression decisions.

So much has been achieved these past 2 years. The innovations briefly described here are now firmly established standard practice. Many of the innovations have already been adopted by other courses within my institution, representing interprofessional educational practice, and this expansion is ongoing. Some (e.g., the Objective Structured Clinical Examination model) have been implemented internationally, with local expansion currently under negotiation. Our use of Google Apps preceded the institutional-level adoption of this technology and has resulted in a recent peer-reviewed publication. This dispersion is a direct result of my continued engagement in HMI courses, in both Boston and Australia.

My work inspired through the HMI has also directly led to my professional advancement. I was formally promoted to manage medicine assessment across all four undergraduate medical programs – a direct result of my successful innovations – and more recently I was promoted to director of medicine admissions, and of assessment data. I also received my faculty's prestigious Dean's Award for Teaching Innovations (2011) to honor this work, and I now sit on university-level assessment committees.

My present sense of community and belonging represents a stark contrast to the professional isolation I felt prior to this engagement. I am eternally grateful for all that I have gained from my involvement with the HMI, from the professional networks and collaborations to the many friendships now formed. All have significantly enhanced my work and the work of my institution. I have a deep and renewed commitment to quality health professions education, and a now clearly defined professional purpose.

Reality Checks

It is always a good idea to build in "reality checks," both for continuous improvement of the HMI program and to step back and reflect on whether my hopes became a positive reality. Just recently, in 2011, the Josiah Macy Jr. Foundation asked for a retrospective and independent evaluation of the HMI programs from inception through 2010. With over 3000 alumni scholars worldwide and 2000 active e-mail addresses an independent, external evaluator (SJB Evaluation and Research) collected both qualitative and quantitative data. This study, conducted over 9 months, provided valuable data from over 600 respondents.

The report concluded there is strong evidence that the combination of attributes that make innovation possible (including, and maybe especially, perseverance!) can lead to very positive results. Nearly 75% of respondents in the Educators and Leaders courses (and 64% in the newer Systems course) felt their HMI experience was personally transformational. The evaluator found that what contributed to such meaningful change were the excellence of the faculty, the pedagogy, and learning about issues faced by health care professionals from other institutions and other countries. Becoming part of the HMI community was extremely meaningful, with close to 80% reporting that meeting new colleagues across a broad spectrum of disciplines was critical to their learning. Close to *95% of survey respondents would recommend the HMI course* they attended to a colleague, and three-quarters would strongly recommend it. In seeking my "reality check," this high rate of enthusiastic recommendation is extremely fulfilling.

Learning Along the Way

It takes time for faculty from different disciplines and schools (even when all are part of the same university) to learn to teach together. In the first and second year of HMI, each faculty member needed to sit in on each other's classes just so we could all determine what each had to offer and how each person's material related to the others. It appears to take at least 3 years to build a cohesive faculty team-teaching approach – in fact, the longer the better.

Every time we wanted to introduce something new to the HMI, such as journal clubs, we would typically have to call it an "experiment" for a year – "let's just test the idea and see if it is well received." There needs to be an engine of new ideas for the courses – listening to Scholars and alumni faculty is the best engine. My extensive travel and involvement in many disparate networks is also a very big plus. I see ideas in other fields and countries and try to think about how they could be connected to our work. You can learn something from everyone in every setting.

Surprising

One personal point of learning deserves emphasis: how hard this new work is in our usual academic culture! Academia is *not* a great "petri dish" for innovation. Internal academic structures can create unexpected barriers. But I was encouraged by constant positive feedback – from studies, from individuals, and from institutions. Hearing from our community members has supported my continued enthusiasm for this work. The fact that 75% of those in our alumni network feel transformed by our courses is the evidence we all need to keep taking risks and implementing more innovations, consistent with our core principles.

Challenges

At this point in the life cycle of the HMI, a major challenge is keeping such a large group of individuals invested and engaged in the faculty and alumni/ae communities. This work takes enormous personal time. I am connected 24/7, as is Terry Cushing, HMI's program manager, to address the issues of the community members. Whether positive comments or queries, both take time and most people expect almost instant answers because that has been our tradition. Transitioning to the better use of social media is a current challenge. Some faculty and alumni are not ready for it and others are. We are figuring out how to create the right balance. We are constantly recruiting (Scholars and faculty) and building courses. That is a 12-month job – there is no academic holiday in this work.

Future
• • • • • • • • • •

In *The Innovator's DNA: Mastering the Five Skills of Disruptive Innovators*,[1] Dyer *et al.* provide their research on the common qualities and skills that exist among innovative leaders. In creating the Institute and in the design and teaching of its courses, we have lived all of the behaviors that make up the "DNA" which (unlike regular DNA) can be created (no laboratory required!). It is fascinating to see that these five skills sound very much like those used by scientists to make discoveries.

Those skills, paraphrased here, are (1) *associating*, which is the ability to make surprising connections across areas of knowledge; (2) *questioning*, which allows innovators to break out of the status quo and consider new possibilities; (3) *observing*, so that innovators detect small behavioral details that suggest new ways of doing things; (4) *experimenting*, in that they relentlessly try on new experiences and explore the world; and (5) *networking* with individuals from diverse backgrounds so radically different perspectives are gained. The authors argue that the five competencies can be learned and mastered. This is good news indeed, since these competencies are an integral part of what the HMI teaches and are also part of our faculty model to help facilitate personal transformation and innovation in health care institutions worldwide.

Innovation with Staying Power

Richard S. Nowakowski, PhD
Randolph L. Rill Professor and Chair
Department of Biomedical Sciences, Florida State University

When I arrived at Florida State University (FSU) a little over a year and half ago, I was delighted to begin to work closely with Myra Hurt, currently a professor of biomedical sciences and the senior associate dean of research and graduate programs at the FSU College of Medicine. Most important for me, as a newcomer, was her deep knowledge of FSU and the research scene in Florida. She is always able to answer my questions and provide the background that made me understand the system. My initial impressions of her were that she had great competence and insight. Later, I realized that my impression fell woefully short of her true leadership abilities.

The moment of realization came when I attended the Harvard Macy Institute course on Innovative Leadership in Medical Education, run jointly by the Harvard Medical School and the Harvard Business School. Myra was one of the instructors, which came as no surprise to me. What did impress me, however, was that no fewer than three of the presenters showed us slides of the FSU College of Medicine educational system for its medical students to illustrate how a truly innovative medical curriculum looks. I knew already that the creation of a new medical school was Myra's student project when she first attended the Harvard Macy Program and that it was her leadership that led to the birth of the FSU College of Medicine. What I realized from the presentations that I heard in Boston was what an impact her "child" has had on the rest of the United States and the world. I say the world because the Harvard Macy Institute attracts an international audience from around the globe. Myra's examples and writing have shown the way to others and, although the FSU College of Medicine was the first new medical school in the United States in 25 years, over 20 additional medical schools have been started in the past 10 years. Myra served as the first chair of the new medical school group when it formed a few years ago! There is no doubt that her leadership stimulated, at least in part, this burst of activity.

References

1. Dyer JH, Gregersen HB, Christensen CM. *The Innovator's DNA: Mastering the Five Skills of Disruptive Innovators*. Boston, MA: Harvard Business School Publishing; 2011.
2. www.harvardmacy.org
3. Armstrong EG, Barsion SJ. Creating "innovator's DNA" in health care education. *Acad Med*. 2013 Mar; **88**(3): 343–8.
4. Rogers CR, Freiberg HJ. *Freedom to Learn*. 3rd ed. Columbus, OH: Charles Merrill Publishing; 1994.
5. Christensen CM, Grossman JH, Hwang J. *The Innovator's Prescription: A Disruptive Solution for Health Care*. McGraw-Hill; 2009.
6. Collins J. *Good to Great and the Social Sectors: A Monograph to Accompany Good to Great*. HarperBusiness; 2011.
7. Armstrong EG, Doyle J, Bennett NL. Transformative professional development of physicians as educators: assessment of a model. *Acad Med*. 2003; **78**(7): 702–8.
8. Christensen CM, Armstrong EG. Disruptive technologies: a credible threat to leading programs in continuing medical education? *J Contin Educ Health Prof*. 1998; **18**(2): 69–80.
9. Armstrong EG, Barsion SJ. Using an outcomes-logic-model approach to evaluate a faculty development program for medical educators. *Acad Med*. 2006; **81**(5): 483–8.

3

Facilitating the Effectiveness of Medical Teachers

Improving Teaching through Faculty Development

Kelley M. Skeff and Georgette A. Stratos

Introduction

This is a story of success built on the commitment of many people – including mentors, teachers, trainees, and institutional leaders – to one another and to a common goal: the improvement of medical teaching. As codirectors of the Stanford Faculty Development Center for Medical Teachers (SFDC), we have had the good fortune to work in the field of education, often receiving the gift of teaching from others, and ultimately being able to pass that gift on to medical teachers around the world.

In the following pages, we offer a narrative about our faculty development program on medical teaching, highlighted by principles that guide our work, our philosophy of education, and comments from faculty who have trained with us. Finally, we discuss the sources of gratification that have continuously enriched our lives for the past 3 decades and our vision for a next chapter in this work. We hope that this story will inspire those who are committed to enhancing their impact as educators/teachers.

Background: The Stanford Faculty Development Center's Clinical Teaching Program

How We Started Our Center

The SFDC was established in 1985 to assist medical faculty to improve their teaching. The Center is the culmination of a collaborative venture that began when we met in 1979 while completing our PhD programs. We recognized the potential for synergy given our differing talents, a common set of humanistic goals, and joy from working with others.

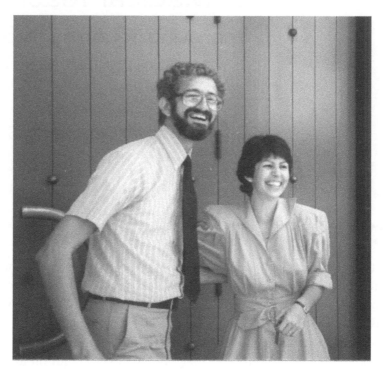

PHOTO 1 Kelley Skeff and Georgette Stratos at the "Stanford Barn" – the home of the Stanford Faculty Development Center (Palo Alto, 1987)

I met Kelley in 1979 while we were both working toward our doctoral degrees (mine in educational psychology from UC Berkeley and his in education from Stanford). Kelley needed help in developing and implementing a rating scale to analyze video recordings of clinical teaching for his dissertation study of attending physicians. With my background in the sociolinguistic analysis of communication skills and education, I seemed to be a natural fit.

My prior work had given me a firm foundation for shifting into the field of medical education. My doctoral research on misunderstandings in everyday conversations between children and adults heightened my appreciation of the influence of contextual factors on interpersonal interactions. A second project – set in the outpatient clinic of the Palo Alto Veterans Administration Medical Center – was a study of the linguistic correlates of successful doctor-patient communication. This work opened my eyes to the highly complex nature of communication in this setting.

As we began working together, Kelley and I gained an appreciation for the similarities in our philosophies (and senses of humor) and shared empathy for the difficulties associated with teaching in the medical setting. Our complementary styles and backgrounds led to the formation of a strong partnership that has persisted over time.

—Georgette Stratos

Originally, the process began because I enjoy teaching. Like so many, I had the desire to share with others whatever I had the benefit of knowing myself. This drive was augmented by being in the field of medicine where the lessons learned had the excitement of science combined with the sensitivity of humanity. Therefore, I entered my fellowship with the goal to show the importance of the role of teaching, committing oneself to successful learning of others.

My plans changed in the midst of my own evolution. My initial thought was that I would be most useful by emphasizing the process of teaching medicine in a manner that would bring attention to the noble role of teaching in academics. However, with the encouragement of mentors, I developed the desire to have a better understanding of the process of teaching and its implementation by others. So my own desire shifted from a focus on the teaching of the content of medicine to the similarly exciting study of the process of teaching. The content changed, but the love of analyzing the process remained. Also, in that evolution, my focus on teaching shifted from a focus on the individual trainee in medicine to the faculty – teachers who would enable many trainees to become more effective physicians. Thus, assisting faculty in medicine became the focus of my work. Although not clear at that time, my desire was to have clinical teachers gain a better understanding of the process in order to more consistently enjoy the gratification of assisting others to learn.

—Kelley Skeff

In 1985, we received a Department of Health and Human Services, Health Resources and Services Administration grant to create a train-the-trainer program that would disseminate a faculty development course on clinical teaching to primary care physicians across the country. This approach would allow us to touch an expanding cadre of teachers, building on a course we developed and implemented locally in 1981 with support from the National Fund for Medical Education. Although our center has created faculty development courses in a variety of subject areas – End-of-Life Care, Geriatrics, Medical Decision Making, Preventive Medicine, Professionalism – in this chapter, we will focus on the Clinical Teaching Program. It is the longest-running program and can be considered the core, embodying the principles on which all the other programs were based.

> I believe the most important lesson from our work and the work of other faculty developers has been the increased recognition that teaching is a complex and challenging process that requires ongoing attention to consistently achieve a high level of excellence. This recognition was clear to a few people in the early 1950s. However, I believe it took 40 years and the work of many people to bring a more general acceptance of this belief. It is also important to recognize that this goal is still not fully accomplished. The recognition of the importance of educational innovation and the usefulness of providing education for teachers in higher education remains challenging. It will probably take another 25 years for teaching improvement to be embedded in the activity of all faculty members as part of their professional development.
>
> One of the most challenging parts of this work has been the ongoing need and search for funding. Education remains one of the most difficult academic tasks to quantify and support. Dedication, the cognitive activity of teaching, and quality teaching time is hard to quantify and therefore financial support is challenging. We were extremely fortunate to be the beneficiaries of a variety of institutional, philanthropic and national funding organizations, including the American College of Physicians; John A. Hartford Foundation; Robert Wood Johnson Foundation; Josiah Macy Jr. Foundation; Pew Charitable Trusts; Shenson Family Funds; Stanford University School of Medicine; and the Veterans Administration. Without these sources, the benefits of our program to faculty could have not been realized. Therefore we are extremely grateful for their support. Our financial needs were satisfied in an ongoing way by moving from supporting organization to supporting organization. The timing of our work was perfectly in sync with the funding for faculty development in primary care as well as the ongoing and enhanced recognition of the need for scholarship in education.
>
> *—Kelley Skeff*

Description of the Clinical Teaching Curriculum

The "Clinical Teaching" course was designed to achieve three major goals: (1) enhance participants' versatility as teachers, (2) enable them to use a seven-component educational framework to analyze teaching, and (3) provide a forum for collegial exchange about teaching. The program incorporates a variety of instructional methods including didactic presentations, group discussion, review of video reenactments of actual teaching interactions, role-play application exercises, and personal goal setting. The formal presentation of the 14-hour course occurs in seven 2-hour interactive sessions. The course is ideally suited for small groups but it can also be delivered to larger groups, using breakout sessions for small group interaction.

Once we received Health Resources and Services Administration funding, our first step was to solidify the core content and instructional methods used in this course. We embarked on an extensive review of the literature on teaching and learning to refine the educational framework that is the touchstone of the course. This framework encompasses the following topics:

- Learning Climate
- Control of Session
- Communication of Goals
- Promotion of Understanding & Retention
- Evaluation
- Feedback
- Promotion of Self-Directed Learning.

For each of these topics, we developed "mini-lectures" that introduced principles of effective teaching along with specific-related teaching behaviors. We produced a set of video vignettes – reenactments of actual clinical teaching interactions – that would stimulate analysis of teaching through the application of concepts introduced in the didactic presentations. We created role-play scenarios and structured a role-play debriefing format that would enable participants to practice teaching in front of their peers in a safe environment, and then identify plans for changing their teaching in the future.

Evaluation of this program has shown that it is highly effective in improving teaching performance across several settings (inpatient, outpatient, lectures) and across all seven educational categories. Using conservative estimates, at least several thousand medical teachers – both faculty and residents – have participated in versions of this course. Evaluation data consistently shows that this experience has been perceived to be useful.

The core content of the curriculum has been stable and robust over the years. Yet, we have continually made modifications to it, adapting the course for delivery to additional audiences (e.g., medical residents as teachers, basic science teachers, surgical educators, pediatricians, psychiatrists, geriatricians, teachers of social work). Revisions reflect new challenges in medical education and our desire to continuously enhance the instructional methods embedded in the course. We made these adaptations to broaden the potential outreach to assist as many groups as possible.

> My initial hope was that this work would benefit people all along the education chain: the teachers, their students, and patients they care for. The course was intended to offer medical teachers a powerful educational experience that not only would give them a conceptual/cognitive tool for improving their teaching across the span of their career, but also encourage them (even challenge them) to question their assumptions about their roles and methods as teachers. If a teacher adopted a systematic and comprehensive cognitive tool (the educational framework) and a motivation to experiment with different teaching approaches, the seeds of behavior change would be sown.
>
> —*Georgette Stratos*

Stephanie Call, Virginia Commonwealth University (2001)*

I continue to live, eat, and breathe the Stanford framework for clinical teachers. I have so much fun running seminar after seminar and working with my chiefs and faculty members daily, incorporating the framework as an assessment tool of teaching. It is truly what gives me greatest pleasure in my professional life.

Note: *Year that the faculty member attended the Stanford Faculty Development Center for Medical Teachers Clinical Teaching Program.

Eugene C. Corbett Jr., University of Virginia (1987)

After 25 years I continue to benefit from and work to further disseminate an understanding and application of the Stanford Faculty Development Program's clinical teaching skills framework. It truly reflects the universal elements of the teaching and learning process. I have no doubt that the seven-component clinical teaching skills framework will remain an enduring, applicable and user-friendly model for advancing the clinical teaching skills . . . of anyone who chooses to further their abilities in education whether at the bedside, in the classroom or in a hallway conversation.

Educational Principles and Philosophical Biases Underlying the Clinical Teaching Curriculum

The drive to make this educational intervention powerful enough to be consistently effective across a variety of teachers and cultures led us to make curricular decisions based on educational principles. Each of these choices also reflects our shared philosophical biases. In this section, we will highlight the key educational principles underlying the choices made.

Respect for Course Participants

Underlying our work is a strong sense of empathy and respect for the medical teachers who participate in our course – their background (which generally does not include training in teaching) and their distinctive characteristics (academic, scientific, skeptical, self-reliant). Faculty participants in our courses come with a great many strengths and characteristics that must be addressed in designing an effective teaching improvement method for them. To have achieved their positions, these faculty members are intelligent. They have mastered difficult content, experienced challenging learning situations, and in many cases, overcome great hardships. Medical teachers, like other adult learners, often base their current approaches on powerful past experiences. They come with a large amount of experience with the educational system, having been students for many years. Given the apprenticeship model of medical education, they also have been teachers, commonly responsible for teaching near peers and colleagues (e.g., interns teaching medical students, residents teaching interns, fellows teaching residents, and faculty teaching all levels). Their experiences with teaching (both as teachers and as learners) can lead to strong beliefs about teaching and learning. They have come to rely on the wisdom of experience as the major guiding force for their teaching methods.

We also recognize the highly challenging nature of their task – teaching an ever-increasing and changing medical content (spanning knowledge, skills and attitudes) in a wide range of settings (from the analogue of a one-room schoolhouse with multiple learners at different training levels to didactic presentations to one-on-one interactions at the bedside). Medical teachers, both clinical and basic science, face a complex teaching task. We believe faculty development must prepare these teachers to face this complex environment, effectively drawing upon their own past experience, principles of education, and an expanded variety of teaching methods. This led to our goal to show respect for the background and contributions of every participant in our course.

The Value of Multiple Instructional Methods

We have included a number of instructional approaches in the course not only to maximize the impact of the training on participants' knowledge, skills, and attitudes but also to demonstrate teaching versatility – one of the stated objectives for course participants. The sessions incorporate approaches that are both teacher-centered (e.g., lecture, guided discussion) and learner-centered (e.g., articulation of personal teaching goals). In addition, we have designed the course so that the facilitator models the effective use of all seven educational categories taught.

Providing a Cognitive Tool for Reflection about Teaching

To help teachers analyze and improve their teaching, we offer them a structured framework with which they can reconsider previously used approaches and consider new teaching behaviors to try. This framework is comprehensive and practical (analogous to the review of systems used by physicians to work up a patient), allowing teachers to recognize what they see intuitively about their teaching and to recognize what they may not see. In addition, by reviewing aspects of teaching in a systematic fashion, participants may discover or redis-cover the underlying basis for their own commitment to teaching.

Nonprescriptive Approach

We believe that all teachers must be in charge of the decision-making process while teaching, since they have a unique perspective about the issues they are facing. In addition, as products of the medical education system, physicians have been taught to be decision makers, relying on their knowledge and experience to make judgments. Therefore, a principle of our method of faculty development is to provide alternative approaches and teaching behaviors, while empowering teachers to decide which ones they wish to use and when they wish to use them.

> Because my educational background did not include medical training, I wondered how I would be accepted by the audience we had targeted for our course. When I started, I felt like a sponge, absorbing all I could about clinical teaching and the particular people we'd be teaching in our courses. I benefited greatly from observing hundreds of hours of hospital teaching rounds and clinic teaching interactions, as well as many discussions with informants. Kelley was an invalu-able guide during this time. As I grew into the work and received feedback, I learned that the perspective I brought could have complementary value to med-ical teachers.
>
> —*Georgette Stratos*

Added to this is our acute appreciation that the complexity of teaching makes it difficult or even impossible to generate specific prescriptions for how to teach that will be valid across learners, content, contexts, and teachers. We strive to avoid the dogmatic stance that there is a "best" way to teach. Given this, our goal has been to teach principles and practices of effective teaching gleaned from educational theory, empirical studies, and practical experience from which course participants can choose, utilizing their own ingenuity. Our intent is to encourage teachers to embrace a spirit of experimentalism and innovation with teaching, expanding their repertoire of approaches to the teaching process.

> Another surprise was the recognition that fully trained faculty may naturally review the teaching of others with a negative, critical eye. Because of our background training, it has been common for medical teachers to review the videos reflecting the teaching of others with a critical perspective rather than a positive one. Physicians are taught to find the problem and try to fix it. Therefore, it has been important to develop methods that enable others to review the activities of colleagues recognizing not only the problems but also the successes of others.
>
> —*Kelley Skeff*

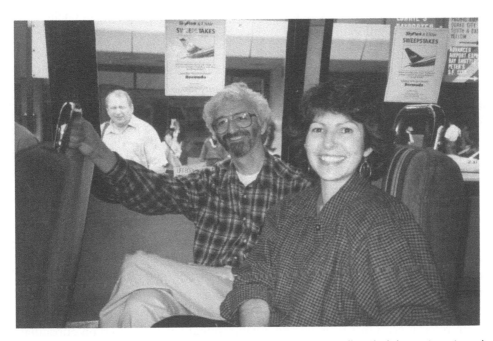

PHOTO 2 Kelley Skeff and Georgette Stratos on the road, expanding their impact eastward and beyond (Colorado, 1995)

Description of the Facilitator-Training Program in Clinical Teaching: Extending Outreach through Dissemination

Having developed, implemented, and tested a method to improve clinical teaching, our goal was to enable others to deliver this course at their own institutions. We designed a monthlong, facilitator-training course to prepare medical faculty to become facilitators of the Clinical Teaching curriculum with sufficient competence/confidence in the prerequisite knowledge base of educational content, grounding in the philosophical basis for the curriculum, and facilitation skills in handling small group dynamics. Only six trainees are selected from among the candidates who apply each year. The intensive program is run on an annual basis and follows a rigorous daily schedule. Major training activities include:

- receiving a curriculum just as participants will receive at home
- reading and discussing background literature related to the curriculum
- reviewing and practicing curricular components, focused on mastery of the content knowledge, teaching process, and philosophical slant underpinning the curriculum
- practice teaching the course to local audiences of faculty/residents, with feedback from SFDC staff
- attending talks by guest speakers from Stanford School of Education
- attending home-site implementation sessions preparing trainees for challenges likely to be faced upon re-entry to their institutions.

In 1986, we conducted our first Clinical Teaching Facilitator-Training program. This program has been offered annually ever since. By the end of 2013, we will have trained 169 faculty to deliver the teaching improvement course to medical teachers at their home institutions. They come from 10 countries and 96 different institutions, including half of the medical schools in the United States (*see* Figure 3.1). These trained facilitators represent a wide range of departments (including internal medicine, pediatrics, psychiatry, surgery, obstetrics and gynecology, family medicine, radiology, anesthesiology, emergency medicine, osteopathic medicine) and the full spectrum of prior teaching experience (from less than 1 year to over 25 years).

Faculty trained as Clinical Teaching facilitators have played key roles in meeting faculty development needs nationally and internationally. Some have taken their training at Stanford as a jumping-off point for further training in the field of education, including advanced degrees. Many have taken on administrative leadership roles at both institutional and organizational levels focused on curricular design/reform, program evaluation, teaching assessment, and learner assessment.

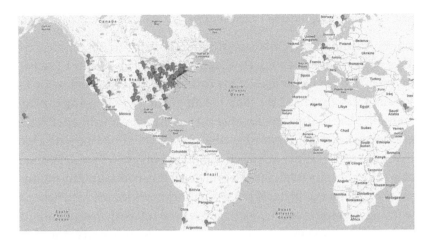

FIGURE 3.1 Location of Home Institutions of Graduates Completing the Stanford Faculty Development Center for Medical Teachers Clinical Teaching (this map comes from Stanford University's Stanford Faculty Development Center for Medical Teachers website and was created using Google maps and mapalist)

Carol Storey-Johnson, Weill Medical College of Cornell University (1995)

I would certainly say that participating in the Stanford Faculty Development Program in 1995 clearly opened the door for dialogue about the importance of teaching at my institution and resulted in "instant credibility" for me personally to achieve my goals in climbing the administrative ladder in medical education. I have given a yearly offering of the Stanford Faculty Development Program Clinical Teaching course for a master's program in the Division of General Internal Medicine through the Weill Cornell Graduate School of Medical Sciences since 1998. It is always rated highly and the learners all seem to have a new view of teaching when they leave the course.

One of the remarkable outcomes of this program is its longevity. For over a quarter of a century, both novice and experienced medical teachers have used this course to advance their knowledge and skills of teaching, reexamine their beliefs about teaching, and rediscover the joy of the teaching process. We believe this success is a consequence of deliberate choices made during the initial planning for this facilitator-training program to tailor a program that would match the backgrounds, abilities, and needs of physician educators.

Glenda Westmoreland, Indiana University (1997)

In 1997 my mentor, Chris Callahan, encouraged me to "go and get some credentials." The Stanford Faculty Development Center for Medical Teachers (SFDC) elevated me in the eyes of my colleagues – they looked to me for advice and I like that I had the tools to help them. Prior to going through the training, I had the love for teaching but not the science to be an effective clinical teacher and mentor to other educators. SFDC armed me with a tool kit that gave me versatility as a teacher. It helped my professional advancement at the university level since I was better able to communicate my own personal goals and was better at self-evaluation. It helped me with national networking. At retreats and the Society of General Internal Medicine annual alumni reunion, I was able to reconnect with others immersed in the SFDC and this always stimulated new ideas. The SFDC has given me the tools to develop and assess curricular products. These skills have clearly enabled me to grow into my leadership roles in geriatric education.

Sandy Valaitis, University of Chicago (2005)

With the information I learned from the Stanford Faculty Development Program in Clinical Teaching, I was also able to develop a new evaluation form for faculty teaching that incorporated more objective measures of their teaching efforts and better documentation of their teaching strengths and weaknesses, which assisted with their promotion. Since completing the course I have been able to share my knowledge with other departments and at other institutions. I have presented workshops at national meetings (Association of Professors of Gynecology and Obstetrics), been invited to be a faculty member of our institution's MERITS (Medical Education, Research, Innovation, Teaching, and Scholarship) fellowship program, and have been recognized by my institution as a Fellow of the Academy of Distinguished Medical Educators. I am deeply grateful for the training I received at the Stanford Faculty Development Center for Medical Teachers.

Educational Principles and Philosophical Biases Underlying the Facilitator-Training Course

In this section we describe some of the educational principles and philosophical biases connected to the durability of this facilitator-training course.

Placing an In-House Resource for Faculty Development at an Institution

An on-site resource can be of great benefit to an institution trying to meet ever-increasing faculty development needs. The institutional investment of training a facilitator offers a mechanism for continuity and long-term support for teaching improvement.

Using Peers as Trainers

Research from the field of diffusion of innovations suggests that innovations are more effectively disseminated by individuals who share similarities with the potential adopters.[1] Therefore, we decided to train medical faculty as facilitators of our teaching course. We designed the monthlong training program so that faculty who had not studied education would gain sufficient background knowledge and facilitation skills to feel confident delivering a course on teaching to peers at their home institutions. This approach has been highly effective overall, and in particular for achieving the third major goal of our course, enhancing collegial

---

Debra Litzelman, Indiana University (1990)

Indiana University School of Medicine (IUSM) has trained or recruited a cadre of Stanford Faculty Development Center for Medical Teachers (SFDC) facilitators. Since IUSM is the only medical school in Indiana with nine campuses, the impact of the SFDC has been statewide. Tangible evidence of the impact of the SFDC on IUSM's academic culture is the growing use of a shared vocabulary (e.g., "learning climate" and "means goals" heard in everyday conversations). Additionally, the seven SFDC educational categories are included in teaching evaluations completed by all medical students throughout the state and by residents within the department of medicine to evaluate their medical educators. Faculty members' teaching summaries reflecting the seven SFDC educational categories are included in faculty teaching profiles used for departmental annual reviews and are also included in faculty dossiers used for promotion and tenure decisions.

I am grateful to Kelley and Georgette for committing their professional lives to systematically affecting the process of medical education throughout the world. They have done this with science, rigor, and faithfulness to the education framework that has held up under the test of time and across cultural differences ... and they have done it with genuine caring and nuanced coaching for each individual educator whom they have trained ... always modeling effective teaching with grace and humor!

---

exchange about teaching. In-group membership gives facilitators a unique perspective on their own institutions' culture and educational environment that can be an advantage for conducting home-site faculty development programs.

Using Explicit Criteria for Selecting Trainees

Our selection of trainees from among the faculty who apply to our program is heavily influenced by two factors: (1) level of individual commitment expressed by the candidate for assuming a faculty development role and (2) evidence of institutional support for the trained facilitator and for faculty development activities. Our aim is to lay a firm foundation for trained facilitators to be successful when they return home and add a new facet to their careers.

Embodying the Educational Principles and Philosophical Approaches Taught in the Teaching Improvement Course while Training Facilitators

We have designed the facilitator-training curriculum to reflect the same principles and philosophical underpinnings that form the foundation of the 14-hour Clinical Teaching course. We believe that by demonstrating the effective practices that the trained facilitators will eventually teach to their colleagues, we provide strong examples for them to follow.

Introduction to the Field of Education

Beyond preparing trainees to disseminate the teaching improvement course, we have constructed the training month to include broader exposure to the field of education. Among other activities, this exposure takes the form of reading and discussing literature from education, medical education, and educational psychology; talking with guest speakers whose academic careers are in education; and brainstorming sessions to explore research interests in medical education.

Charles Rohren, Mayo Clinic (1992)

Georgette's session on educational philosophies, the readings of Carl Rogers,[2] and Kelley's modeling of humanistic teaching opened my eyes to the truth for me that "It's not what teachers do, but how they feel about students that creates healthy places where children can grow."[3] Throughout the month in Palo Alto I was aware of these conditions in my interactions with Kelley and Georgette. It is a debt that can only be repaid by passing the insights along to my learners and colleagues by creating those conditions that facilitate learning. By being . . . a teacher. Thank you.

T. Robert Vu, Indiana University (2003)

The Stanford course has made me a much more mindful teacher – I use the framework to analyze my own teaching. What may work one day for one team or one set of learners doesn't necessarily translate to the next set of learners. Mindful practice is a key enabler of versatility and the Stanford course has helped me to achieve that.

Attending to the Power of the Intervention

In addition to these factors behind the successful dissemination of this program, we must return to the power of the 14-hour teaching improvement course itself. Unless the method has perceived value to the target audience, the dissemination approach will matter little.

Craig Cheifetz, Virginia Commonwealth University, Inova Campus (2000)

The experience while at Stanford was nothing short of amazing. Having trained over 150 faculty and more than 300 residents at my institution, perhaps most meaningful was the comment of a 30-year veteran gastroenterology physician who said, "I took this course because I felt bad for you and wanted to make sure you had enough participants, but having taken the course it was the best learning experience I have had in 30 years!"

Larry Greenblatt, Duke University (1997)

A senior, nationally recognized teacher attended one of the first Clinical Teaching courses I taught at Duke. At the first session, he seated himself in a chair right next to me and acted as a cofacilitator. After three or four sessions he returned to our class this time sitting across the table with the other faculty. He spoke about his astonishment when he tried some of the teaching strategies that I was encouraging my participants to try. He found them to be not only effective, but also a lot of fun. For the remainder of the workshops he returned each week with great excitement to talk about the adventures he was having teaching in ways he had never thought about before.

Next Chapter in Our Story

Further International Expansion of Our Work

> From the start, our goal was to disseminate this training broadly, beyond our own institution – first nationally, then internationally. We were intrigued by the question of whether the training would have value to cultures beyond the original one we targeted (US primary care faculty).
>
> —*Georgette Stratos*

> Once I shifted my goals to helping faculty, expanding the breadth and generalizing the impact and faculty across many institutions became an important goal. Thus, the process shifted again from knowledge of the essential aspects of education and teaching to the mechanism for dissemination of this essential knowledge and skills to others around the country and around the world.
>
> —*Kelley Skeff*

We are excited about the potential to nurture the seeds already planted in different cultures by presenting workshops for new groups of teachers and by training additional facilitators from international sites who can serve as long-term, in-house faculty development resources. Our international experience to date has given us multiple opportunities to study the universal value of the approach we've adopted. Trained facilitators have implemented the program in a variety of countries in Europe (Sweden, Switzerland, Germany, and Russia), Canada, and South America (Chile, Argentina). In addition, in recent years, we have traveled to Asia (China, Taiwan, Japan) and to countries in the Middle East (Saudi Arabia, Qatar, United Arab Emirates), often accompanied by alumni trained at the SFDC, to introduce the training at institutions eager to provide faculty development for

> One surprise has been the robustness over time and populations. Both the Clinical Teaching and the Facilitator-Training courses have stood the test of time and cross-cultural exposure. Although we have continually refined them, the core of each of these programs is recognizable 25 years later.
>
> —*Georgette Stratos*

their teachers. So far, it appears to be effective across these cultures. These experiences continually rekindle our motivation and inform our practice as faculty developers.

> Probably the most satisfying and gratifying portion of this endeavor was the recognition that the principles of education and educational psychology for medical teachers reflected the principles for human learning across national cultures. The recurrent recognition of the importance of a positive emotional environment for teaching and learning has been gratifying, as that was a key part of what we wanted for all learners. We also saw repeatedly that faculty across the world respond both to a respectful environment as well as an intellectually challenging and gratifying structure.
>
> *—Kelley Skeff*

Carlos Reyes, Pontificia Universidad Católica de Chile, Santiago (2003)

I did the Stanford Faculty Development Center for Medical Teachers Clinical Teaching course 7 years ago. Coming back to Santiago, Chile, I started giving the course to attendings at Pontificia Universidad Católica de Chile Medical School. Soon I was invited by our Faculty Development Center to give the course to teachers from across the country, not only physicians but also nurses and dentists. At the moment there are 129 participants in 15 courses. At the same time I have also been training residents at Pontificia Universidad Católica de Chile Medical School. Today 93 of them have completed the course and the results of the evaluation are really encouraging. I can tell you that this is the first initiative to give formal clinical teaching training to residents in Chile.

Jeff Wong, Medical University of South Carolina (1992)

Hungarian author, playwright, and poet Frigyes Karinthy's[4] short story "Chain-Links" introduced the concept of "six degrees of separation" to the world, sometimes referred to as the "human spider web." In the field of medical education, the impact that the Stanford Faculty Development Center's (SFDC) program in Clinical Teaching has had on this discipline is so widespread that an analogous "Medical Education Clinical Teaching spider web" would contain even fewer degrees of separation connecting all of the world's medical educators.

> Taking the SFDC's concepts "on the road" to various institutions and meetings in the United States as well as across cultures, to Russia, Spain, France, China, and Singapore (helping to enhance connections within the human spider web) has been life changing for me. I have seen firsthand how the educational struggles of teachers in all of these countries are nearly identical – and how the SFDC model can be successfully transported across different cultures and medical education systems to touch the soul of those educators in Kazan, Lyon, Pamplona, and Hangzhou, as they strive to improve their abilities to teach effectively. At a recent international faculty development conference in Toronto, Ontario, I met an educator from Ulan Bator, Mongolia. I had never met anyone from Mongolia before but as we started chatting, it was evident why she wanted to meet me: she had heard about my work using the SFDC in China and she wanted to find out more about it. The medical educator "chain-link" is growing.

Enhancing the Relevance of Our Teaching Materials

We are in the process of updating the video vignettes used to stimulate discussion about the educational principles taught in our course, developing scripts selected from video recordings of teaching interactions in surgical (e.g., operating room and tumor board sessions) and clinical teaching settings (e.g., in hospital wards and internal medicine clinics), reflecting the current settings and challenges for teaching medicine.

Training a New Generation of Facilitators and Providing Booster-Training

Our intent is to extend the network of trained facilitators, by training a "second generation" of facilitators who will continue to assist medical teachers around the world. We now regularly receive applications from faculty who could be considered our "grandchildren" – that is, faculty who have attended programs offered by previously trained facilitators at their home sites who now want to take on a faculty development role themselves. Another goal is to offer refresher training to previously trained facilitators as a means to boost their motivation for this type of work and to provide them with updates on the training.

Conclusion

In conclusion, we have had a gratifying opportunity to be able to assist committed teachers around the world to discover new horizons in their careers as teachers and find new insights into their own philosophy and love of teaching. It has been our honor to play a role in helping medical teachers enhance their impacts on those whom they teach. Moreover, we feel privileged to help others redefine their core values as members of the helping professions.

Door

It opened today
I felt it swing wide
With a gasp
An Exhalation
A sigh of relief.

I did not even know that I had closed it.

It opened today
And my soul poured out
On paper
With a whisper,
A breath of freshness.

I had forgotten that I needed it.

It opened today
My emotions leaked
On my face
With a tear,
A first ripple of the tide.

I had ignored the call of the sea.

It opened today
And I feel strangely
Cleansed
Anointed
A washing of soul.

I had missed the purity of thought.

It opened today.

—Donna Ray, MD

Note: Written September 5, 2002, after playing the teacher in the Communication of Goals role-play that Georgette facilitated for the 2002 Geriatrics in Primary Care facilitator-trainees. Reproduced with permission.

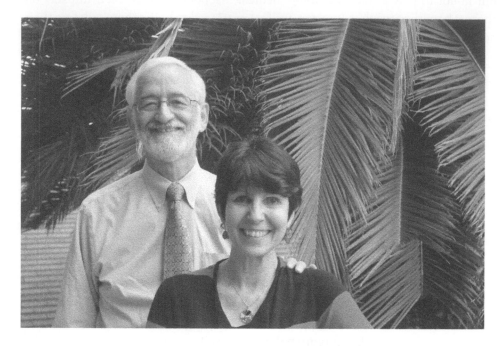

PHOTO 3 Kelley Skeff and Georgette Stratos – still working and smiling together after all these years (Palo Alto, 2012)

References

1. Rogers EM. *Diffusion of Innovations.* New York, NY: Free Press; 1962.
2. Rogers C. *Freedom to Learn: A View of What Education Might Become.* Columbus, OH: Charles E. Merrill Publishing; 1969.
3. Combs AW. *A Personal Approach to Teaching: Beliefs That Make a Difference.* Boston, MA: Allyn & Bacon; 1982.
4. Karinthy F. "Chains" or "Chain-Links" (depending on translation), a chapter in *Everything is Different.* Hungarian publisher unknown; 1929. Translation reprinted as "Chain-links" in chapter 2: Historical developments. In: Newman M, Barabási A-L, Watts DJ. *The Structure and Dynamics of Networks.* Princeton, NJ: Princeton University Press; 2006.

4

Education of a Teacher

William T. Branch Jr.

IN 1982 I WAS DIRECTOR OF THE BRIGHAM'S PRIMARY CARE RESIDENCY Program. I had recently published the first edition of my textbook *Office Practice of Medicine*.[1] Completing the book had been stressful. I needed a rest and I imagined attending the Task Force, now the American Academy on Communication in Healthcare, on the Medical Interview's first course would be relaxing. Yet, I was a skeptic. Beyond asking open-ended questions, what was there to learn?

The course was like a circus with exciting new ways of teaching but also great upheavals as self-designated titans of medical interviewing struggled for leadership and recognition. There were "touchy-feely" sessions in the afternoon. I skipped out on these. But I learned useful techniques in our small group of four matriculants who worked with a facilitator in the mornings. I learned to make empathic, supportive, and reassuring statements. So simple, and yet transforming. During the following year, I incorporated empathy and support into interactions with my patients. Patients expressed gratitude. My attitude toward practicing medicine had previously been that it was a strict discipline, requiring intense concentration, and long hours of work, and was not meant to be personally rewarding. Now, practice felt rewarding, not only because patients expressed gratitude but also because my support and empathy seemed to be therapeutic for them. I was doing much more good for my patients and felt better about myself.

The next interviewing course was in California. Now, the "touchy-feely" part was simplified into an unstructured group with just a few rules: among them, maintain confidentiality and speak for yourself. The basic idea was to give and receive honest feedback in a safe environment. This opportunity for genuine interactions with my peers was far more appealing to me than the previous year's "sensitivity exercises." However, I had no idea the extent to which this group would influence me. Since then, I have been in and facilitated many groups. I have seen individuals gain insights, address inhibitions, and even have epiphanies, but never have I experienced a group as powerful as this California one. My momentous discovery was fully experiencing the benefits of giving and receiving emotional support. These were people I knew. The experience was real and not constrained by the structure of me being "the doctor" and the other being "the patient." Whereas previously I had learned skills that transformed my practice, the California group reached me on a different level. I wanted other doctors to learn what I had experienced – the immensely therapeutic power of providing support and understanding. This became a calling.

I had embarked on a journey with a remarkable group of people. Looking back, I think we were sometimes naïve and overly idealistic. Nevertheless, I credit many who became lifelong friends also with being teachers, colleagues, and fellow travelers along a journey that became my life's work. This was a joint effort. I will mention or quote from some special folks who worked with me but I could never express enough gratitude or even find space to quote from all who contributed along the way.

In Providence, I vividly remember meeting Mack Lipkin Jr. We were walking across the green in front of dormitories at Brown University when Mack introduced himself. I clearly recall standing behind Penny Williamson as we waited to be served seafood at an outdoor dinner. Sam Putman was in my small group. Rosalind Mance was the facilitator. Julian Byrd and Steve Cohen-Cole developed the three-function model. I could name dozens of others whose interactions were important to me from this course experience, but space does not allow.

By serendipity, a huge opportunity presented itself. Dean Daniel Tosteson began the New Pathway at Harvard Medical School, a radical new curriculum with a major component addressing patient-doctor relationships. The New Pathway had many mothers and fathers, who contributed to important aspects of it. My part spans the years 1985–1995. My friend Bob Lawrence was instrumental in choosing me to be one of four group-facilitators for the pilot "Patient-Doctor Course." This course was another eye-opener. "Patient-Doctor" used participatory, small-group methods. Though the course was controversial, I witnessed medical students enthusiastically embrace this world of learning around what I now know as medical humanism. I assumed a leadership role as director of the third-year component. Later on, a crisis developed over lack of small-group facilitators. My contacts with many clinicians enabled me to assist in ensuring that we had sufficient numbers. Then, there was need to improve the clinical skills component. Offered that job, I embraced it. I believed that this course was the single most important educational initiative of the New Pathway. The dean then decided to generalize the New Pathway project to all Harvard medical students, but did not include the Patient-Doctor Course. Several of us and most students advocated strongly on behalf of the course. The dean then approached me with barely a month's notice to organize a curriculum for a new, required first-year course. This was to be the largest required course on patient-doctor relationships that had ever been mounted. It was an unprecedented opportunity to benefit the medical students. The challenge was exhilarating. We quickly formed a group of faculty to organize the required First-Year Patient-Doctor Course.[2] Within 2 years, we took an even more unprecedented step by instituting a required Third-Year Patient-Doctor Course.[3] The concept of having all students leave their clinical clerkships to address the human dimensions of medical care was radical. Initially, resistance in the third-year was strong from clerkship directors and some medical students. Convinced that I was right, I persisted in advocating for our approach. Within a year, the students had embraced our new course, largely because of their engagement in the small-group experience. Opposition melted. Third-year "Patient-Doctor" succeeded by creating small-group dynamics that promoted compassion and caring and an attitude of seriousness toward mastering skills to do so.

In planning the curriculum for the first-year course, I made two controversial decisions. The first was to organize the course almost entirely in small groups. Opposition to this decision arose from those who felt that students needed to learn from "experts" in subjects like communication skills and medical ethics. To me, the advantages of small groups, the mentoring and role modeling by carefully selected faculty members, the cooperative learning among the students, and opportunities for them to learn by doing rather than listening to lectures, far outweighed any disadvantages.[4] My other decision was basing the first-year course on medical interviewing. This proved a groundbreaking decision. Never before had this much emphasis been placed on learning to interview patients. However, having students go to the bedside to master skills ranging from basic listening and asking open-ended questions to the conveyance of empathy and support offered huge rewards. It anchored the course in reality. Discussions on alternate weeks explored issues opened up by the patients' stories, which added enormous richness and relevance to the discussions. Furthermore, the students mastered intricate interviewing skills never previously presented in this degree of depth to medical students. Skeptics believed the students would reject medical interviewing, preferring to master the stethoscope. The skeptics were wrong. Bolstered by faculty development sessions, our facilitators proved skillful at leading the small groups. Students took to medical interviewing like ducks to water. They often expressed the belief that "this is why we came to medical school." A most heartening observation made during this time was the high level of skills that some medical students developed. We were discovering hidden talent.

The third-year course was even more groundbreaking. No one previously, to our knowledge, had taken all students off of the clerkships on a weekly basis to focus in small groups on patient-relationship issues. The many colleagues involved in first-year Patient-Doctor were joined by a new team of colleagues ready to undertake third-year Patient-Doctor. It was at that time that I began a most rewarding collaboration: Richard Pels joined our group as curriculum coordinator. Richard and I met regularly and worked out the new Patient-Doctor III curriculum. I attribute many key ideas to Richard, such as our focus on the issues that students encountered during their clinical experiences.

Developing a Patient-Doctor Course for the Third Year of Medical School

Richard Pels, MD
Assistant Professor of Medicine, Harvard University School of Medicine

I had the privilege of working with Bill during the decade of the 1990s as he crafted a new, required "Patient-Doctor III" course for third-year Harvard Medical students. The goals of the course were to provide students with a relevant psychosocial curriculum to complement their daily experience on clinical clerkships and perhaps more importantly, to provide a havened space for critical self-reflection.

Bill confronted substantial challenges in championing this endeavor. Many medical school leaders and large numbers of teaching hospital faculty opposed the Patient-Doctor III course. This was a new course. It pulled students away from their clerkship to be taught by faculty who were often not affiliated with that clerkship. The course content was underrepresented in the third-year curriculum and the teaching method was rarely utilized by the clerkships. Many students expressed ambivalence about the course and some students outright opposed it, for many of the same reasons. In addition, the course proved particularly challenging for the small number of students who were very uncomfortable with explication of the emotional content of their third-year experiences.

Despite these challenges, the course achieved remarkable success. The vast majority of students greatly valued the opportunity to convene each week. The course developed a cadre of talented, loyal faculty facilitators who increasingly came to value the ways in which it added meaning to their professional lives. And it provided a space for curricular innovation that simply did not exist elsewhere in the third-year curriculum.

As the course director, Bill exercised essential leadership for this endeavor through role modeling, persuasion, academic dissemination (in the form of publication and local, regional and national workshops), and mentoring of junior faculty. Underpinning Bill's success with this remarkable project was his advocacy for an idea founded in personal reflection on years of experiences as a clinician-educator. Bill provided clarity of purpose and a single-minded tenacity, coupled with an uncommon ability to listen to and incorporate other points of view.

The Patient-Doctor III course no longer exists in the form so strongly advocated by Bill. I regard the disappearance of the course as proof of its ultimate success, as the passing years have seen greater ownership of this curriculum by the teaching hospitals and transformation of the students' often fragmented third-year experience into a more continuous relationship with one faculty and one hospital. We had always felt strongly that this content would be most effectively taught through more immediate connection to students' clinical experiences, by the faculty supervising them, at the site where these experiences happened. But decades of observation had taught Bill this wouldn't happen reliably through encouragement or cajoling. The teaching hospitals would need to be shown the essential nature of this curriculum and they would need to be persuaded by the students. The students served as remarkable ambassadors. And Bill encouraged them to share their reflection papers at every opportunity, so their written word in essence became a powerful change agent. What was once considered a radical threat to the students' clinical education is now understood as an essential component of an outstanding clerkship. Students continue to convene with trusted faculty in continuous small groups for havened reflection. And many of today's faculty were students during the initial innovation! The lasting impact of this innovation is testament to Bill's remarkable vision, passion, and collaborative leadership style.

It was Bob Lawrence who suggested use of the critical incident reflections[5] alluded to earlier. These short vignettes became a backbone for reflective learning in the course. Students wrote from the heart. They shared with us amazing stories of their experiences and their incredible perspicacity as they observed the behavior and actions of residents and faculty members. Some behaviors were good, some were bad. As Dean Tosteson said, "When you turn over a rock, the bugs may run out." But, we learned how students experienced the clerkships, their feelings and their amazing insights.

Our qualitative analyses of critical incidents revealed the extent to which students identified with patients and resisted socialization into medicine's "hidden curriculum."[6] This challenges the notion that empathy erodes during the clinical years. Given a strong third-year Patient-Doctor Course, we saw amazing empathy.[7] Another key concept applied to the moral development of medical students. Using Kohlberg's theories,[8] students could be viewed as progressing from the conventional group morality of adolescence to postconventional adult-morality based on moral principles. But then, potentially, they regressed as the hidden curriculum pressured them to move toward a new group morality. Patient-Doctor was a countervailing force. Further analysis identified a major theme of their ethical dilemmas as related to the ethics of caring based on Carol Gilligan's theories.[9] Caring and wanting to care fit best with the experiences and dilemmas faced by medical students on the wards.

Harvard's Third-Year Patient-Doctor Course

Gordon Harper, MD
Associate Clinical Professor of Psychiatry, Harvard University School of Medicine
Succeeded Bill Branch as director of the third-year course

In developing the New Pathways Third-Year Patient-Doctor Course, Bill identified several things that were needed.

1. *Reflection, reflection, reflection:* including validation of experience and validation of learning from experience.
2. *Off-site time and space:* away from the clerkships physically, with protected time, and away psychologically from the urgency and pressure of immediate patient care.
3. *The curriculum that is necessary but that no one ever quite gets to . . .:* ethics, communication, spirituality, diversity, quality improvement, prescribing – topics all would agree doctors need but that never get included in the clerkship schedule.
4. *Academic standing:* in medical schools that pride themselves on academic standing, the Patient-Doctor Course had to be a course, not just a socialization group.
5. *Connections:* hence, the longitudinal nature of the course – a year, even though later chipped away.
6. *Writing:* we learned that written reflections, shared with a small group, meant a great deal to the students. We didn't know at first what gifted writers we would find.

Lessons from Patient-Doctor like those that Gordon Harper describes led me to recognize educational principles that have remained germane to my career as a medical educator.[10] Use of experiential learning alternating with reflective learning was the method that I found effective in shaping skills, values and attitudes of the learners.[11,12] Reflective learning in these settings focused on professional, not personal, issues. Group-process added to the power of the learning, because the group provided support, assured participants that they are not alone in facing dilemmas, provided its own role models, and created its own learning climate, a kind of counter to the negative aspects of the hidden, or informal curriculum.[11,12]

Participants in the learning groups remained sensitive and highly committed to norms, like empathy, compassion, moral courage, and honesty. We recognized these as group norms.[12] The process at the personal level was often transformative. Our large-scale educational interventions also impacted the culture of the institution, making it more humanistic.[2,3,9] These were powerful lessons. I have applied these lessons subsequently; although I feel that much potential has been lost as interventions on this scale with this much focus on medical humanism have yet to be adopted by many medical schools. Nevertheless, thanks to many dedicated teachers and practitioners over the years, medicine as a whole has made steady progress. There are new curricula now at many medical schools that incorporate some or most of these principles.

By the mid-1990s, I had reached a point of seeking new challenges. Our courses had achieved a pinnacle, and others could carry them forward. We had also reached a pinnacle in the primary care residency at the Brigham. We had wonderful teachers and leaders to carry this effort forward. I was convinced that only by continuing education in the human dimensions of medical care, such as what we had done with the medical students at Harvard, into residency training and even faculty development could we succeed in truly improving the educational environment. Backsliding occurred at every level unless the educational process continued. This was my theory. I looked for a way to apply it by becoming division director of general internal medicine at Emory University. Here, I would have the ability to mentor faculty who in turn could influence medical education on a higher level.

We created a successful primary care residency program at Emory. Having the primary care residents off the wards and working with us for 1-month blocks enabled them to focus on learning communication skills and to write critical incident reports. Qualitative analysis of their reports revealed three phases of the residency experience. The initial few months was "formation of identity" – a time when residents asked, "Why did I become a doctor? Who are my role models? What type of doctor will I be?" This benign phase was superseded by what we called "descent to the depths." For the next nearly 2 years, the residents faced a real possibility of burnout. Their stories revealed the immense stress, the sleep deprivation at that time, and most powerfully, the pain and sadness of losing patients. It was this "failure to cure" that seemed most discouraging. I remembered feeling the same deep frustration with my inability to benefit terminally ill patients admitted one after another during my own internship. However, the final 6 months of residency were marked by "reconciliation and renewal" – a time when residents realized their relationships with patients were beneficial, patients expressed gratitude, and residents looked forward to the next phase of life. Educational implications of our observations include emphasizing guidance at the beginning, support in the middle, and more guidance and reflection at the end of residency.[13] We could do this in our small, primary care, residency program where we controlled the 1-month blocks. Another implication seemed clear to me. The graduating residents were poised for rapid professional and personal growth. They were leaving the residency's hidden curriculum, and many were joining the faculty. Perhaps faculty development provided the key to achieving a more humanistic medical culture.[11,12]

What kind of program could most benefit the faculty? How could we develop their capacities as humanistic role models to the point that they would change the "hidden curriculum"? A group of us formed at an annual interviewing course in Worcester, Massachusetts, to work on humanistic teaching of faculty. I suggested we become a permanent group to identify and study methods for humanistic faculty development. We called this "The Humanistic Group." Some of the original folks have continued with this project, while many others have joined. We began with workshops, and elicited ideas and insights from participants' stories. We published a paper on the concept of teaching the human dimensions of medical care,[14] and other papers on outpatient humanistic teaching.[15,16]

A small grant from the Schwartz Foundation enabled a study of faculty role models.[17,18] I sought a larger grant from the Arthur Vining Davis Foundations to put into practice an ideal faculty development program. This would be a longitudinal program done in small groups that would, again, utilize the methodology of experiential learning alternating with reflective learning in the context of a supportive group process. Our group included experienced facilitators from five medical schools. We devised a written curriculum and selected eight promising teachers at each school to meet twice monthly in small groups for a period of 18 months. I believed this to be the ideal faculty development program to achieve genuine, even transformative, positive changes in humanistic role modeling and teaching.

Thomas Inui and Richard Frankel joined with me in devising the evaluation. With much guidance from Tom, we created the Humanistic Teaching and Practice Evaluation questionnaire, which was later validated at Indiana University.[19] The questionnaire filled out by learners compared our faculty participants with controls. Results revealed a powerfully positive effect of the intensive longitudinal faculty development process. All ten items on the questionnaire and the questionnaire as a whole statistically significantly favored the participants. All five schools favored the participants. At Emory, we were able to show that overall teaching evaluations, as well as gender, age, and specialty did not account for the differences.[11] Although there is always the possibility of selection bias, the strong results suggest a genuine positive outcome.

Faculty Development in Humanism

Richard Frankel, PhD
Professor of Medicine and Geriatrics, Indiana University School of Medicine

One of the things that I admire most about Bill is that he embodies what he is passionate about – and that is humanism. Working through the complexities of working with five sites, developing a curriculum that could be adjusted to fit a range of institutional contexts, collaboratively developing curricula and instruments to measure impact takes a special set of skills. Bill is a master at creating "safe space," whether it is for students and residents to talk about what is meaningful in their training or their lives or for a group of faculty to come together around how best to teach and evaluate humanism at the bedside. He is also able to pass along his knowledge and wisdom about teaching humanism as evidenced by the fact that the curriculum succeeded at every site and was not dependent upon a single charismatic individual.

Another example of practicing what you preach occurred recently when Bill invited a group of us to prepare a workshop entitled Fostering Professional and Humanistic Development in Young Faculty Members: The "TEACH" Program, Faculty Development to Enhance Medical Humanism, for the annual scientific meeting of the Society of General Internal Medicine. During our initial planning calls for the workshop, we discussed presenting the process we had used in developing and implementing the curriculum along with outcomes from the five sites that participated in the study. There was some enthusiasm for this approach but several faculty said that it seemed like "the same old, same old," and wasn't likely to raise the level of the audience's enthusiasm or motivation to use the curriculum.

With Bill's guidance, we decided to give workshop participants an "immersion" experience by offering three different mini-versions of the curriculum that participants could sort themselves into by their own level of interest: using narratives based on appreciative inquiry; giving feedback; and being and becoming a role model. The mini-sessions were highly interactive and meaningful. At the end of the workshop we asked participants if they cared to share in the larger group what their experience in their group had been.

One mid-career faculty member said that she had actually been feeling burned out for some time and a little lost in terms of her direction and motivation for doing medical education. In the session on being a role model she was reminded of a note she had received recently from a resident she had taught a decade ago. The resident was writing to say that the faculty member had been an inspiration to her in her training and continued to be to this day.

Having shared the story in her small group, the faculty member was able to recapture how good it felt to be valued, and how revitalizing this was and also how surprising it was given the fact that she didn't remember that she had done anything "special" for this particular resident during her training. She went on to say that a big, new insight from the workshop experience was that you never can predict what effect you may be having on others, or when you will find out about it. The idea that one is always having an effect, in this case positive, was reason for hope, renewal, and a few tears of joy for this faculty member. It was a stunning self-disclosure in front of a large audience and an equally stunning insight that the faculty member took away from being "immersed" rather than lectured to about the curriculum. The bottom line was that the kind of safe space that Bill is so good at creating among the faculty responsible for delivering the curriculum was re-created in the workshop. It also reproduced the same kinds of experiences that participants at each of the sites were having in the longitudinal curriculum.

One form of intelligence in medicine is based on the pursuit of objective, unbiased knowledge and evidence. Another form of medical intelligence is based on wisdom, curiosity, and engagement in affairs of the heart as well as the mind and body. Both types of intelligence are necessary to practice clinical medicine and both can be approached with equal rigor. Bill is the rare individual whose intelligence in both the biological (read his textbook *The Office Practice of Medicine*[1]) and the humanistic aspects of medical care come shining through as a beacon of inspiration and wisdom for others.

Developing Capacities for Humanism in Faculty

Peter Weissmann, MD
Associate Clinical Professor of Medicine and Endocrinology, University of Minnesota School of Medicine

It is with great pleasure that I think back over the time I have come to know Bill. I first remember meeting him at a national meeting of the Society for General Internal Medicine. He was facilitating a workshop for clinician educators. Although I remember few details of that meeting, I do remember thinking as I left that I had met a wise, kind, and erudite man who was doing the kind of work that I aspired to do.

Our next meeting, also serendipitous, was at the national meeting in Atlanta of the American Academy on Communication in Healthcare (AACH), then called the American Academy of Physician and Patient. Bill was the senior facilitator for my small learning group. During a Balint group exercise, I presented the case of Jack, a young man under my care for a severe traumatic brain injury, whose health was deteriorating rapidly for no clear reason. I'd found myself in several difficult encounters with Jack's mother. She looked to me for hope in the face of her son's illness, but – feeling powerless – I could not honestly offer any. Bill helped me refocus my attention to the care that I could provide Jack and his mother even if he would not recover. Instead of dreading my next encounter with them, I went home looking forward to it.

We met again a year later at the next national AACH meeting in Worcester, Massachusetts. This time, Bill and I found ourselves in the same self-selected project group that would meet for the duration of the weeklong course around the topic of "teaching humanism at the bedside." I recall being very excited that several senior and well-known Academy members, Bill among them, had chosen to participate in this group. Here Bill showed me the difference between a good physician and a visionary. Whereas I would have been satisfied to present something of interest to the rest of the conference participants at the end of the week (and then stop), Bill's vision was much greater. Ten years later, thanks largely to Bill's initiative and guidance, our group is still at work. With the help of several large grants (that Bill has helped us acquire), we have been able to create training programs at over a dozen American medical colleges to foster what we call the human dimensions of care. We have published a good number of papers about this topic in highly regarded medical journals and presented at numerous national medical meetings.

Along the way, I have also served with Bill on the AACH Executive Committee and the AACH Board of Directors. I'm not sure Bill has understood to what degree he has mentored me by his example, his kindness, and his support. He has shown me how to thoughtfully revise an academic paper and how to present at academic conferences. He has come to my home institution as a visiting professor. He has written to support me as I have sought new professional challenges. Whatever success I have enjoyed in medicine, both academic and clinical, I owe in large part to Bill's mentorship. It has been my great fortune to know Bill, and I feel deeply blessed by our association and friendship.

Peter's comments in particular capture a lesson learned along the way. I had started out in the early 1970s believing that medicine was an intellectual pursuit. Thanks to working with wonderful colleagues such as those whose comments have been included in this chapter, I later fully realized and incorporated the belief that relationships count the most, both in doctoring and in one's career.

Aim High: The Emory Faculty Group

Kimberly Manning, MD
Assistant Professor of Medicine, Emory University School of Medicine

The most pivotal moment in my career took place in 2004 when Bill asked me to join him in a faculty development group focusing on medical professionalism and humanism. In these sessions led by Dr. Branch, we received instruction on reflective writing as a tool for teaching and processing clinical experiences. With his encouragement, I revised and submitted a narrative I wrote during our faculty development for publication. It was Dr. Branch who told me to "aim high," and much to my delight, my manuscript was accepted to the first place I sent it – *JAMA*. This planted a seed in me that grew into what is probably my greatest career interest: reflective writing as a means of teaching professionalism and humanism in our learners. Since that initial spark, I have had three publications accepted in the *Annals of Internal Medicine*, two publications in *JAMA*, and another in *Academic Medicine*. Under his guidance, I have presented several workshops on Reflective Writing in Medicine at national meetings, at both the Department of Medicine and School of Medicine faculty development programs and as a part of the curriculum for students in the School of Medicine.

When I started a medical blog focusing on medical reflections in 2009, it was Bill who encouraged me the most and who viewed it as something of great potential. That simple idea is now featured every week on the *ACP Hospitalist Blog* and *The Health Care Blog* and was even chosen by *O, The Oprah Winfrey Magazine* in 2010 as one of "4 Medical Blogs You Should Read Now."[20]

Last spring, I led a fourth-year medical student elective on reflective writing, and I currently have four manuscripts in process with medical students interested in narrative writing. I am certain that I never would have considered any of this were it not for the constant validation, support, and examples set by Bill. When I sat down to write this, I asked myself a simple question: Where would my professional career be were it not for Dr. William Branch? The answer is simple – nowhere even close to where it is today. Thanks to Bill, I have found my passion and my voice in medicine – something many clinician educators spend an entire lifetime trying to locate. Now that I have, I am better at the things I do, I teach with more zeal, I mentor others with more passion, and I have become fearless when it comes to educational innovation.

Therefore, it was especially rewarding for me to facilitate my own Emory faculty in a group enrolled in our humanistic faculty development project. Participants were all members of my Division, whom I chose because of their promise as young faculty teachers. They were compared on the evaluation to some of the other star teachers in our program, who were of similar age and background. Their results on the Humanistic Teaching and Practice Evaluation questionnaire were significantly positive for the group, but of much more importance to me, the group as a whole developed an enormously cohesive commitment to the human side of medicine. We had adopted appreciative inquiry narratives as the vehicle for reflective learning. This component was extremely influential on their development.

Learning to Teach Humanism

Lisa Bernstein, MD
Associate Professor of Medicine, Emory University School of Medicine

The Faculty Development in Humanism Project was transformative for my teaching. Dr. Branch personifies the humanism he works tirelessly to impart to his faculty, medical students, and residents. As the mentor of our group, he introduced us to rich techniques to employ for our own introspection. While I considered myself fairly empathic prior to participating in the Humanism group, the discussions with Dr. Branch and my colleagues about various ways to teach and model humanistic treatment of patients tremendously impacted my future educational endeavors and clinical practice. I have subsequently incorporated many of these reflection techniques into my bedside and classroom teaching and this experience directly affected my professional development as a clinician-educator, as well as my personal growth.

Since finishing the faculty development project, I have progressed well along my career path. I became codirector of the Becoming a Doctor Course and leader of one of the four student Societies in the new curriculum instituted in the Emory School of Medicine in 2007. Working with Dr. Branch as my codirector, I have incorporated into curriculum patient-centered interviewing, empathic communication, and other elements of humanism in medicine that I learned from the faculty development program. In addition, I was promoted to associate professor and I have been fortunate enough to win several prominent local, regional, and national teaching awards.

We embarked on a qualitative study of the narratives collected at Emory. The Emory group had continued to meet for 5 years. The Emory participants were my coauthors and were participants-observers of the process, which added their keen insights to the qualitative analysis. They identified three phases of their work in faculty development: the initial year focused on becoming empathic physicians; the second year focused on role modeling empathy and compassion to learners; and the remaining years focused on their development as "empathic leaders," a

---

Finding My Passion

Stacy Higgins, MD, FACP
Associate Professor, Emory University School of Medicine

Arriving at Emory as a new faculty member in 1999, I knew that I enjoyed teaching but I didn't know how to focus my efforts, or how to make teaching into something that would advance my career. Sitting in Bill's office one day, he asked me a question that in retrospect seems incredibly simple, "What do you like? What are you passionate about?" With that prompt, I went on with his support to found the women's clinic at Grady, as well as to initiate the women's health curriculum for the Internal Medicine residents. This allowed me to mesh my clinical interests with a need to participate in the educational program, and made me the local expert on topics such as contraception, menopause, and the intersection of medicine and gynecology. I have used this expertise to lecture to health departments around the country, educating countless practitioners on the care of the female patient. Without the vision and support of my mentor, I would not have had the time to develop the curriculum, start and maintain the clinic, or teach others on the topic.

This is just a small example of Bill's guidance of my career. He has been an unwavering supporter of me in my role as director of the Primary Care Residency program. He assists with recruiting, hosts dinners for the residents, promotes the program at national and international venues, was instrumental in my Health Resources Services Administration grant proposal and award, coauthors papers with me, and nominates me for committees and awards, both local and national. He does this completely unselfishly, because he wants to see me grow and succeed, and much of it is done behind the scenes without any recognition. Everyone should be so fortunate to have someone like Bill Branch in their corner, cheering them on, encouraging them to reach for the next goal and to dream of bigger things. I am very thankful that I do.

term they coined. Their personal and professional growth was spectacular.[12] As I look at this group today, including those whose comments appear in this chapter, I am struck with admiration for their achievements: an assistant dean and vice chair of education for the Department of Medicine, director of the Primary Care Residency Program, director of the Transitional Residency Program, associate director of the overall Residency Program, society leader and course director for the Being a Doctor Course in the New Curriculum at Emory Medical School, winners of numerous Golden Apple Awards, the Herbert W. Waxman Award for Medical Student Education given by the American College of Physicians, and the Papageorge Award – the highest teaching award given at Emory University School of Medicine.

Being a Division chief definitely provided the opportunity to mentor and thereby foster the growth of young faculty members.

Unquestionably, the success of the faculty in our division has been my greatest personal reward. Meanwhile, the work of the Humanistic Faculty Development project has continued. Eight new schools joined a second grant and are now completing the evaluation of their results. I can relish the potential contributions of the many participants (almost 100 to date) in this project. I also think back on our many primary care residents at the Brigham as well as at Emory. Also, there were hundreds of Harvard medical students who took the Patient-Doctor Courses. Their influence affects an ever-widening circle of future generations in medicine.

The next phase of the faculty development project hopes to include an additional expansion to new schools and more detailed studies of the impacts of the participants in the program on their learners.

Medicine is truly and fully a human experience. There is no more idealistic endeavor on the planet. We adopt science as the best pragmatic method for benefiting people, but the human side of medicine should always be paramount.

In this chapter, I have acknowledged some special people who worked with me in my career. Many others contributed to my development. There were mentors, projects, and phases of my career that I could not address due to space limitations. And, legions of doctors work in the trenches to cure the sick and alleviate suffering. We are all privileged to be part of this endeavor.

Reflection and Take-Home Points

What would I say to young physicians who want to be medical educators? I should place my comments in the context of today's environment, much different from when I began my career in the 1960s. I should imagine what it is like for someone starting out now. The pathway that I followed in a different time may or may not be applicable to today.

- First, if education is your passion, by all means follow it. I heard advice, even as recently as the 1990s, that a career in medical education would be a dead-end. In my view, this is profoundly wrong-headed advice. No one should choose a career trajectory based on external markers of success. Choose the career that will give you personal satisfaction.

- Recognize what is important and will ultimately provide satisfaction. I believe a great source of professional satisfaction is your relationships with your learners. You will enhance their success the most if you care about them, develop strong relationships with them, and are supportive in all ways. I wish I had thoroughly learned this lesson early in my career.

- Seek training in teaching and education. Fellowships are available and valuable. For those who missed the opportunity to take a fellowship, there are faculty development programs and part-time programs for learning in medical education.

- My next advice was a constant theme in this chapter: Find as many friends and collaborators who share your passion for education as you can. Success in education requires a joint effort. At the end of the road, friendships will prove of lasting importance.

- Find a mentor. Surprisingly, mentoring was not much talked about in my early career. Some lucky people had mentors. It was a hit-or-miss situation. Today, mentorship is recognized as a key to success. So, if you are a young person starting out, develop mentoring relationships.

- At times, you may have to stand up for your principles or battle for your beliefs. As long as this is for the ultimate good, and not a struggle for self-aggrandizement, you should engage in this struggle. But in fighting, do not burn your bridges. Try to keep good personal relationships even with those who disagree with you.

- Finally, one truth remains a constant through time, the point I made in the beginning: It is the people and the relationships that matter most at the end of the day.

References

1. Branch WT Jr., editor. *Office Practice of Medicine*. 4th ed. Philadelphia, PA: WB Saunders; 2003.
2. Branch WT Jr., Arky RA, Woo B, *et al.* Teaching medicine as a human experience: a patient-doctor relationship course for faculty and first-year medical students. *Ann Intern Med.* 1991; **114**(6): 482–9.
3. Branch WT Jr., Pels RJ, Harper G, *et al.* A new educational approach for supporting the professional development of third year medical students. *J Gen Intern Med.* 1995; **10**(12): 691–4.
4. Branch WT Jr. Notes of a small-group teacher. *J Gen Intern Med.* 1991; **6**(6): 573–8.

5. Branch WT Jr. Use of critical incident reports in medical education: a perspective. *J Gen Intern Med.* 2005; **20**(11): 1063–7.

6. Branch WT Jr., Pels RJ, Lawrence RS, *et al.* Becoming a doctor: critical-incident reports from third-year medical students. *N Engl J Med.* 1993; **329**(15): 1130–2.

7. Branch WT Jr., Pels RJ, Hafler JP. Medical students' empathic understanding of their patients. *Acad Med.* 1998; **73**(4): 360–2.

8. Branch WT Jr. Supporting the moral development of medical students. *J Gen Intern Med.* 2000; **15**(7): 503–8.

9. Branch WT Jr. The ethics of caring and medical education. *Acad Med.* 2000; **75**(2): 127–32.

10. Branch WT Jr. The road to professionalism: reflective practice and reflective learning. *Patient Educ Couns.* 2010; **80**(3): 327–32.

11. Branch WT Jr., Frankel R, Gracey CF, *et al.* A good clinician and a caring person: longitudinal faculty development and the enhancement of the human dimensions of care. *Acad Med.* 2009; **84**(1): 117–25.

12. Higgins S, Bernstein L, Manning K, *et al.* Through the looking glass: how reflective learning influences the development of young faculty members. *Teach Learn Med.* 2011; **23**(3): 238–43.

13. Brady DW, Corbie-Smith G, Branch WT Jr. "What's important to you?" The use of narratives to promote self-reflection and to understand the experiences of medical residents. *Ann Intern Med.* 2002; **137**(3): 220–3.

14. Branch WT Jr., Kern D, Haidet P, *et al.* The patient-physician relationship: teaching the human dimensions of care in clinical settings. *JAMA.* 2001; **286**(9): 1067–74.

15. Gracey CF, Haidet P, Branch WT Jr., *et al.* Precepting humanism: strategies for fostering the human dimensions of care in ambulatory settings. *Acad Med.* 2005; **80**(1): 21–8.

16. Kern DE, Branch WT Jr., Jackson JL, *et al.* Teaching the psychosocial aspects of care in the clinical setting: practical recommendations. *Acad Med.* 2005; **80**(1): 8–20.

17. Weissmann PF, Branch WT Jr., Gracey CF, *et al.* Role modeling humanistic behavior: learning bedside manner from the experts. *Acad Med.* 2006; **81**(7): 661–7.

18. Weissmann PF, Haidet P, Branch WT, *et al.* Teaching humanism on the wards: what patients value in outstanding attending physicians. *J Commun Healthc.* 2010; **3**(3–4): 291–9.

19. Logio LS, Monahan P, Stump TE, *et al.* Exploring the psychometric properties of the Humanistic Teaching Practices Effectiveness Questionnaire, and instrument to measure the humanistic qualities of medical teachers. *Acad Med.* 2011; **86**(8): 1019–25.

20. Behen M. *4 Doctor's Blogs to Read Now.* Available at: www.oprah.com/health/Best-Doctors-Blogs (accessed February 3, 2013).

5

Influencing the Culture of Educational Assessment in Academic Health Science Centers

Eric Holmboe and William Iobst

Origins of the Faculty Development Course in Assessment

We appreciate the opportunity to share with you our story about a faculty development course in assessment and evaluation at a very challenging time for medical educators. The catalyst for our journey was simply personal need. Both Bill and I (Eric) have served as program directors in the past; upon starting that job we quickly learned that we did not possess sufficient knowledge and skills in assessment and evaluation. In this chapter, I will start by describing my own journey in developing the course. Bill will provide a unique perspective as an early "consumer" of the course (described later in this chapter) and as the current director of the course at the American Board of Internal Medicine (ABIM). Bill will provide some concluding thoughts about the future direction of faculty development in assessment.

My "aha moment" came when, as a new training officer for a naval internal medicine residency program, I had to sit down with all the residents to discuss their mid-year performance. As I reviewed the traditional monthly evaluation forms that had been completed after each rotation, I found very little useful information related to how the resident was actually performing and that could be used for feedback. Furthermore, almost all the ratings were 6 or higher on a nine-point scale with few to no comments provided. On paper, everyone appeared to being doing "superior" work. I quickly realized that in order to perform effectively as the training officer, I would have to learn a lot more about assessment and evaluation, and use this new knowledge and skill to reform our evaluation system. Thus began my own journey nearly 20 years ago that continues to this day. The difference now is the substantially increased need for better assessment in the context of medical education reform. The educational community is in the middle of a difficult transformation to competency-based medical education (CBME).[1] Simply put, CBME is "an *outcomes-based* approach to the design, implementation, assessment and evaluation of a medical education program using an organizing framework of competencies."[2] The important distinction here is the focus on outcomes – meaning that programs have a high level of confidence, based on robust assessment and curricula, that the graduating trainees can do what the training program says they can do for the benefit of the public. No longer is it sufficient to simply say a trainee has completed the course of instruction. While my examples will be grounded in my US experience, CBME is now a worldwide phenomenon.[2] Box 5.1 provides some examples of terms commonly used for medical trainees at different levels.

Box 5.1 Terms Used to Describe Trainees in Medical Education

Undergraduate Medical Education (Medical School)	Postgraduate Medical Education (Specialty Training)
Medical students	Interns (e.g., typically first postgraduate year in the United States and Canada)
Clinical clerks	Residents (e.g., the United States and Canada)
Subinterns	Foundation trainee (e.g., the United Kingdom)
	Registrar (e.g., the United Kingdom and Africa)
	Senior house officer (e.g., the United Kingdom)
	Fellow (e.g., subspecialty trainee in the United States and Canada)

Over the past decade, policy makers and the public have expressed and directed high levels of frustration at the graduate medical education enterprise. As a result, they are now applying increasing pressure to produce a workforce possessing a set of competencies that can meet the needs of a twenty-first-century health care system. Few can argue that the current performance of the US health care system is optimal. The educational community has to assume some accountability for the current state of affairs. For example, a recent article examining the relationship between the site of training and ultimate practice patterns found a significant correlation between practicing physician obstetrical complication rates and where the physicians completed their obstetrics and gynecology residencies.[3] Another study found substantially low performance on a host of quality measures for the care of the vulnerable elderly among 42 internal medicine and family medicine programs.[4]

Multiple studies over decades have demonstrated that too many students and residents graduate with significant deficiencies in basic clinical skills, core competencies for all physicians. On top of this long-standing situation, programs today must also develop curricula and assessment regarding the knowledge, skills, and attitudes in the newer competencies of evidence-based practice, quality improvement, and systems-based practice. An outcomes-based education system requires a training program to know, with a high degree of accuracy and precision, that trainees are truly ready to transition to the next stage of their careers. This is not possible without valid, reliable, accurate, and effective assessment.

Early Principles

When embarking on any learning journey, *a first principle is to find like-minded colleagues to do the work together.* I was incredibly fortunate to encounter several talented colleagues who shared my interest in assessment. At Portsmouth, Virginia, I partnered with Dr. Rich Hawkins, now senior vice president at the American Board of Medical Specialties, to change the evaluation approaches in the internal medicine residency program. Rich and I literally divided up the various methods of assessment between the two of us, taking responsibility for our assigned evaluation methodologies to teach each other and our faculty colleagues. As we performed this review, we quickly realized that many assessment methods were available, but that we had to choose the best combination of methods and tools to meet the local needs of our own program. This is *a second important principle when implementing anything new within a training program: ensure the change serves the needs of the local training system as well as the needs of the larger public.*

Rich and I were also fortunate to work with Dr. Louis Pangaro, a renowned educator who had developed, along with Dr. Gordon Noel, the "RIME" (reporter-interpreter-manager-educator) framework for evaluating the performance of medical students during their third-year medicine clerkships.[5] RIME was my first introduction to a useful, understandable frame-of-reference for teaching, performing, and coordinating evaluation. The RIME framework enabled faculty to make better judgments about student performance.

Dr. Pangaro provided my first experience in organized faculty development. During my time as training officer, I also served as an onsite medical student clerkship director for the medicine clerkship of the Uniformed Services University of the Health Sciences. As the university-wide clerkship director, Dr. Pangaro led seven sessions on how to be a better teacher. Drs. Georgette Stratos and Kelly Skeff developed these wonderful 2- to 2-and-a-half-hour sessions at Stanford University (*see* Chapter 3). From this early experience and by participating in the intensive monthlong course at Stanford a few years later, I learned that teaching and assessment was a systematic science with empirical evidence and theory to guide effective practice.

Through this experience with RIME and the Stanford faculty development program, I realized the importance of educational theory and research. I became motivated to look outside medicine for evidence to design new assessment approaches and think about different research methodologies to study assessment. As you consider developing faculty development programs, *the third principle is to look outside medicine for helpful evidence and theories.* For example, much of my early work in designing faculty development was heavily influenced by literature from the performance appraisal field[6,7] that highlighted techniques used to improve performance evaluation in other businesses and industries.

Over the next several years, Rich Hawkins and I, working with faculty colleagues, implemented new formative assessments that included medical record audit and feedback, standardized patients using the objective standard clinical examination approach and increased emphasis on direct observation. We felt it was time to share our learning through a workshop at a national meeting. A workshop at a national meeting is a wonderful way to share ideas with colleagues and test out faculty development approaches. In our case, our first 90-minute workshop was a truly helpful "Apollo 13" mission.

While the reviews were generally positive and the participants' comments kind and patient, we learned that trying to get through 90 slides in 90 minutes was not an optimal strategy! *Principle four is to ensure the faculty development activity meets the needs of the audience; which means they need time to interact, manipulate, and reflect on the content to get the most out of the experience.* Be sure to focus on those essentials that enable them to make a meaningful change in their own programs.

The First Course at Yale University

In 1999 the Accreditation Council for Graduate Medical Education (ACGME) formally announced the six general competencies now in common use in the United States and laid out the timeline for the transformation to CBME. Recognizing the importance and value of good assessment and evaluation in CBME, Rich Hawkins and I developed a weeklong course in assessment. We piloted and refined portions of the course via workshops locally and at national meetings. By 2001 we were ready to test the impact of a weeklong course using what we had learned from the science of learning, health services research, epidemiology, and performance appraisal.

We were fortunate to secure a modest amount of funding from the Robert Wood Johnson and American Board of Internal Medicine (ABIM) foundations. This funding enabled us to test the course using a randomized controlled design with faculty from multiple programs. *This fifth principle is vitally important in designing and studying faculty development programs: they should involve multiple sites and programs whenever possible.* As noted earlier, faculty development programs have to meet local needs. Given the substantial heterogeneity of training environments, resources and culture, these contextual differences will have substantial impacts on how faculty development interventions work (or don't) back at the home institution.

Testing faculty development interventions in multiple contexts is therefore essential, and we were very grateful to the Robert Wood Johnson Foundation and the ABIM Foundation for their support. After recruiting approximately 40 faculty participants from among internal medicine residency programs in the Northeast and middle Atlantic states, we randomized them into control and intervention groups. The intervention group completed the weeklong faculty development course with a special focus on direct observation.[8]

The results of the study suggested that a structured, experiential training program could change the quality of faculty observation ratings of clinical skills. The intervention started with the review of several scripted, videotaped clinical encounters with a resident that focused on history taking, physical examination, and counseling. The videos were followed by a mini-lecture describing the scope of the problem in clinical skills and direct observation. The course participants then performed an interactive group exercise that used the techniques of performance dimension (PDT) and frame-of-reference training (FoRT). These techniques helped them develop a set of common criteria, a shared mental model, of what unsatisfactory, satisfactory, and superior performance in clinical skills should be in behavioral terms (*see* Box 5.2). They then used those criteria with the same videotape encounter(s) they viewed at the beginning to see how their ratings changed after the PDT/FoRT exercise.

The course participants spent an entire afternoon practicing direct observation skills, using outcomes of the morning PDT/FoRT exercises, to observe and evaluate a standardized resident interacting with a standardized patient. After one person in the role of the observer/evaluator provided evaluation with feedback to the resident, the small group of peers, with a trained facilitator, provided feedback to the faculty participant.

Box 5.2 Methods to Improve the Evaluation of Trainees

Rater Training Method	Description	Example
Performance dimension training	Familiarize course participants with appropriate performance dimensions or standards to be used in their own evaluation system by reviewing the dimensions of a performance or competency. They then work in groups to improve their understanding of these definitions with review of live performance and videotape.	Course participants discuss the elements of an effective counseling session for a patient starting a new medication for a common medical condition, such as hypertension.
Frame-of-reference training	Course participants practice observation skills with standardized patients and residents performing at various levels of competence. One person provides feedback to a standardized resident. Group discusses evaluation after each "encounter," focusing on reasons for the differences among course participant ratings of the resident's clinical skills.	Course participants watch a standardized resident counsel a standardized patient starting a new medication for hypertension, with the resident performing the counseling at a poor, satisfactory, and superior level in random order. The elements of informed decision making are used to calibrate evaluations and feedback.

Adapted from Murphy and Cleveland[7]

After 8 months, we brought both the control and the intervention participants back to view a second set of scripted, videotaped clinical encounters (nine encounters each for the baseline and follow-up ratings, using a new set of videotapes at follow-up). We found that the intervention participants were more appropriately stringent with reduced range variability on a number of the videotapes compared to the control group.[8]

We were very excited by these results and developed a more practical 2- to 2-and-a-half-hour version for course participants to use at their home institutions using only the videotapes for rating practice after an abridged PDT/FoRT.

Fortunately, two other research groups tried this abridged approach and did not find any changes in ratings. The lack of positive effect using a significantly shorter version of the direct observation training provided valuable insights. One obvious reason was the substantial difference in time and the nature of the training experience – the original study involved 8 hours, including 4 hours of experiential practice with real-time feedback. However, we also realized we didn't really fully understand what were the "active ingredients" that were most important. Perhaps the randomized controlled trial had been premature. We realized that perhaps some pilot tests to refine and improve the faculty development intervention as part of studying "complex interventions" (i.e., interventions that consist of multiple components) might be a worthwhile step. We'll come back to this later, but suffice it to say that evaluation of any faculty development intervention, properly designed for purpose, is a highly valuable endeavor.

The Course, 2001–2011

After learning many lessons from the randomized trial of the weeklong course, we launched our ongoing course in 2001. The course has evolved substantially over the last 10 years as new research about competency-based medical education and assessment has been published and disseminated. The course centers on teaching and skill practice in all the major assessment methods (*see* Box 5.3).

Box 5.3 Assessment Methods
- Rating scales and evaluation forms
- In-training examinations
- Chart-stimulated recall and other methods to assess clinical judgment
- Direct observation (e.g., mini-clinical evaluation exercise)
- Multisource feedback (360-degree evaluations)
- Patient experience surveys
- Simulation and standardized patients
- Medical record audit and feedback
- Evaluation of evidence-based practice
- Portfolios
- Approach to residents in difficulty

In recent years, the course has added workshops on milestones and "entrustable" professional activities, systems approach to evaluation, feedback, and effective functions of competency committees. A milestone simply represents a significant point in development and helps to define the appropriate developmental trajectory of a trainee.[2] An entrustable professional activity, as defined by Olle ten Cate, represents the routine *professional*-life activities of physicians based on their specialties and subspecialties. The concept of "entrustable" means a practitioner has demonstrated the necessary knowledge, skills, and attitudes to be *trusted* to *independently* perform this activity.[9]

One of the favorite workshops among the course participants is a daylong activity focused on improving direct observation skills.[8] The morning session provides the participants with an opportunity to work with the training techniques of PDT and FoRT to develop discriminating criteria (i.e., frame of reference to judge and discriminate between levels of performance) for important clinical skills.

In the afternoon, the participants get a chance to apply the techniques and skills practiced in the morning with live standardized patients and residents. This live practice, with feedback from peers and a facilitator, provides robust hands-on practice experience. For most of the participants, this is the first time they have ever received feedback from colleagues and highlights the importance of participant practice with feedback as part of a faculty development program. This *sixth key principle – emphasize practice with peer feedback – is used throughout the weeklong course*.

We have greatly benefitted from feedback from participants over the years as they work to implement lessons learned from the course into their own program. What follows are some reflections from past participants and course faculty. Uniquely, one of us (Bill Iobst) was an early participant who has now become the course director.

Reflections from the Participants

The success of any faculty development course or program depends on whether it meets the needs of the individuals or groups who participate. Dr. Susan Padrino and Dr. Peggy Stager (both at Case Western Reserve University) attended the course together in 2005. Their reflections on the course and their subsequent work together are provided in this chapter. Over the years we have encouraged institutions to send at least two individuals to the course together so they can work together when they return home. This increases the probability the participants will be able to implement an institutional culture change to their evaluation systems at home. As you will note, there were successes, but there were also things that didn't work or that were not sustained. We think it is important to hear both experiences.

The Importance of Colleague Partnerships

Susan L. Padrino, MD
Medical Director, Douglas Moore Health Center
Assistant Professor, Department of Internal Medicine and Psychiatry
University Hospitals, Case Medical Center, Cleveland, Ohio

My memories of the course and its impact on my academic and clinical life are mixed in with memories of my other major task since then: parenting. I was newly pregnant with my first child when I took the course, so it occurred at a turning point in my life. Since then, I have had three children (and look forward to a new turning point: a life without diapers!). Likewise, the course has borne fruit for me in three major areas.

Immediately after returning from the course, I was filled with enthusiasm and started to apply the methods of assessment and evaluation to our internal medicine resident continuity clinic. In the first few months, we managed to get our preceptors together for two evening sessions to discuss what our standards should be. There was a flurry of activity: documents were created, e-mails were exchanged, and the conversation really got going. We even agreed on a process for using the mini Clinical Evaluation Exercise, a tool to rate resident clinical skills, in clinics. Then, I left for 3 months of maternity leave, and the momentum was lost. Without a champion and because of the early stage of the process, the endeavor proved too difficult to keep moving. Unfortunately, there is still a slight (maybe subconscious) attitude among some preceptors that "oh yeah, we tried that and it didn't work." This has made the momentum even harder to recover.

Peggy Stager and I began working on a series of workshops to educate and train faculty in some of the skills we had learned in the course. These included workshops on Direct Observation, Giving Feedback, and the "Problem Learner." There were two crucial elements that made this a successful endeavor. The first was the opportunity to work with an experienced faculty member. As much as we worked collaboratively, Peggy was really a mentor to me. Without the benefit of her wisdom, I doubt these workshops would have developed successfully. I think it was a coincidence that we both ended up at the American Board of Internal Medicine course together, but it turned out to be a fortuitous one. The second crucial element was having an institutional structure on which to "hang out our shingle." At Case Western Reserve University, we have the Center for the Advancement of Medical Learning. Through the Center, we were able to offer courses, collect feedback, and get support with details such as scheduling, attendance, and Continuing Medical Education credit. This allowed the workshops to grow and improve. Ultimately, this has led to dissemination across many departments throughout our health systems (University Hospital, Veterans Affairs Medical Center, MetroHealth Medical Center). Along with Peggy, I have also presented variations of the workshops for podiatry faculty at their national educational meetings.

Beginning a New Personal Journey

Peggy Stager, MD, FAAP
Associate Professor of Pediatrics
Division Director, Adolescent Medicine
MetroHealth Medical Center, Cleveland, Ohio

The content of the program was extremely comprehensive and entailed multiple methods of learning including traditional classroom lectures, dynamic discussions, videos, self-reflection, and group exercises. In addition, Dr. Holmboe designed a day where we attended the testing center. Here we not only performed direct observation of a resident performing a history/physical, but also, in an ironic twist, some of us were then evaluated on our abilities to give feedback. This was a very useful learning experience in that we were videotaped and had the opportunity to see ourselves "perform" as a preceptor. Furthermore, the "resident" gave us direct feedback about our feedback to them. I had never had that opportunity before in all my years as a medical educator. It was a terrific hands-on learning experience that bonded our group.

Once back at our home school, my colleague and I began to plan how we might share all that we learned. We were fortunate in that our school of medicine has a Center for Medical Learning. It was through this center that we were able to "advertise" or "market" our learning sessions to all of the teaching hospitals and departments associated with the School of Medicine. Had it not been for the unique infrastructure and support from the Center, I think it would have been much more challenging to get our proposed workshop ideas out to the general faculty.

Since returning from the program, Dr. Padrino and I have given numerous workshops on topics such as direct observation, giving effective feedback, and the problem learner. In nearly every situation, we learned to tailor the program to the needs of the specific group. We have met with a wide variety of teaching attendings in our region including internists, pediatricians, surgeons, obstetricians/gynecologists, anesthesiologists, and emergency medicine physicians. They have taken back to their departments or training programs what they learned from our workshop. In addition, we have learned a great deal from our colleagues who attended the workshops. This two-way learning experience has fostered a dynamic process in creating and shaping the future training workshops.

In summary, the training session at American Board of Internal Medicine on clinical competencies was the beginning of an interesting journey as a medical educator. It allowed me to bring back to my school of medicine new ideas, new methods, and new materials to share with my colleagues. It pushed me to develop my own materials and continue on the journey of learning. In doing so, the dynamic experience of the workshops and seminars helped shape me as a teacher *and as a learner*. I didn't anticipate that at each and every session as the teacher, I too would be a learner. That has been the greatest lesson of all.

After running the course for 3 years at Yale University, the first courses held at the ABIM were given in collaboration with Dr. Richard Hawkins who was by then working at the National Board of Medical Examiners. It is an example of how one's career trajectory can take interesting turns – 10 years after we met at the Portsmouth Naval Hospital, Rich and I found ourselves again working in Philadelphia, Pennsylvania. The course took advantage of the simulation lab at the National Board of Medical Examiners and allowed us to expand our reach. One of the early participants at the ABIM course was Dr. Christopher Smith from Boston whose interest in the course was precipitated by a new job.

Assessment as Continuous Quality Improvement

Christopher Smith
Codirector, Rabkin Fellowship in Medical Education
Rabkin Fellow in Medical Education
Associate Professor of Medicine, Harvard Medical School

In 2003 the director of the Internal Medicine Residency Program at Beth Israel Deaconess Medical Center (BIDMC), Dr. Eileen Reynolds, invited me to become an associate program director. With the invitation came a special charge: reinvent the residency program's assessment and evaluation programs. I was thrilled to be asked to be an associate program director. It was only a few years prior to this, after being exposed to brilliant and inspiring teachers and discovering a love and passion for medical education while a house officer at BIDMC, that I transformed my career goals. Surely, this passion, along with my educational experiences and training, first as a chief medical resident and then as one of the first members of the new Rabkin

Fellowship in Medical Education at BIDMC and Harvard Medical School, had prepared me for this new challenge. Besides, it was only a matter of assessing the residents . . . how hard could it be? Unfortunately, I would soon get the answer to this question and learn why Dr. Reynolds had this special charge for me – the assessment system in place was barely functional and provided little in terms of meaningful data. After fully recognizing the scope of the challenge of revamping our evaluation system, Dr. Reynolds recommended I attend the American Board of Internal Medicine Faculty Development Course in Evaluation directed by Drs. Eric Holmboe and Richard Hawkins.

The course was rich in content, focusing on assessment tools and skills needed to create an effective competency-based evaluation system, while allowing ample opportunity to solidify these skills through hands-on activities. However, the true value of the course went beyond lectures, simulations, and handouts; it provided me with the confidence needed to redesign our evaluation system and bring about effective change. The course gave me "permission" to try something new, improve upon it, and try it again.

Over time I have come to appreciate that assessment is not something one masters; rather, one must strive to constantly learn from one's learners and colleagues in order to make improvements. As such one cannot accept the status quo, even when there are no readily apparent problems with the evaluation system. With this in mind we now continuously reassess how we teach and assess even the most traditional aspects of medical education. An example is creating novel mechanisms to teach and assess procedural skills, both in live and simulated patients. We constantly strive to create new, more continuous evaluations that assess a variety of educational and quality improvement measures, focusing on direct observation, formative feedback and objective measures.

Over the last several years, with the thoughtful input of many residents and faculty, we have extended the quality and scope of evaluations and have sought to establish a culture that values formative feedback and assessment. At the same time, I have further appreciated the profound responsibility involved in evaluating learners. This responsibility is certainly owed to society to produce competent physicians; however, equally important is our responsibility to the individual learner. Evaluations hold tremendous power and ultimately drive learning. However, evaluations must be handled with care as they can easily damage the fragile confidence of learners of any age. Because of the power and responsibility inherent to the evaluation of learners, the importance of the Faculty Development Course in Evaluation created and directed by Drs. Eric Holmboe and Richard Hawkins cannot be overstated.

Given the breadth of assessment tools and methods, we also recognize how important it is to bring in other expertise and expand the cadre of faculty who can help teach and disseminate the knowledge and skills from the course. We've been very fortunate to work with a number of talented faculty over the years. Two continue to work with the course today. Dr. Michael Green is a general internist at Yale University and an expert in evidence-based practice. Mike has taught in the course almost from its beginnings at Yale, covering the important and evolving field of evidence-based practice assessment. Dr. Jennifer Kogan is also a general internist, currently a faculty member at the University of Pennsylvania. Jen has been intimately involved with the direct observation training, and over the past 2 years has led a large research study at the ABIM on direct observation. Her team's groundbreaking work on direct observation is changing our understanding of how best to train faculty in the critical assessment skill of direct observation.

Faculty Development as a Path to Self-Improvement

Michael Green
Professor of Medicine, Yale Primary Care Internal Medicine Residency Program,
Yale University School of Medicine

Medical educators have long struggled to collect, interpret, and apply evaluation data regarding their trainees. Among the many reasons for this frustration have been deficiencies in the direct observation of trainees' clinical interactions – deficiencies in observing at all and deficiencies in observing accurately. Dr. Eric Holmboe addressed this issue in developing a national Faculty Development Course in Evaluation of Clinical Competence. I have enjoyed teaching in this course for the last 10 years, from the formative workshops at Yale University to the current fully developed weeklong format at the American Board of Internal Medicine. My roles include leading a seminar on evaluating evidence-based practice and facilitating small groups as they practice direct observation of resident-patient encounters in a simulation laboratory.

In the early days of the program, I recall my excitement in seeing the results of rigorous medical education research find application in the training of internal medicine program directors and other key faculty. Dr. Holmboe applied lessons from industrial psychology in developing direct observation of competence training, which includes behavioral observation, frame-of-reference, rater error, and performance dimension training. In a randomized controlled trial, trained faculty were more comfortable with direct observation and rated observations of clinic skills more stringently.

Teaching in this course has definitively helped my small group facilitation skills, refined my own trainee evaluation skills and, with every trip to the American Board of Internal Medicine, renewed my commitment and energy as an educator. In facilitating and debriefing the simulation lab sessions, I discover new ways to engage retiring participants, create the motivating "need to know," and productively give feedback. I return home to my role of preceptor in the residents' continuity clinic with rekindled determination to fit direct observation into an already hectic afternoon. Sometimes I sense a "moral" dimension in the urge to observe. That is, I more acutely feel my responsibility to the patients these residents will care for after they leave this supervised training. I feel less willing to attest to their clinical skills based only on their reports of clinical encounters.

Finally, in recent years I have been struck by the enthusiasm and determination of the course participants. Yes, they represent a selected motivated group, willing to take a week from their professional and personal lives. Nonetheless, as they busily work in small groups, ask provocative questions in seminars, and share their illuminating local experiences, I consistently sense their commitment to improve their programs and the "state of competency evaluation" in graduate medical education.

Confronting our Assumptions and Personal Skills through Faculty Development

Jennifer Kogan
Associate Professor, Department of Medicine, Perelman School of Medicine at the University of Pennsylvania

When I was a medical student, resident, and fellow, direct observation of trainees' clinical skills with patients (i.e., observation of history taking, physical examination, counseling, etc.) was an infrequent, and more often than not, absent occurrence. In fact, I only remember being observed during a patient encounter a handful of times during my medical school Introduction to Clinical Medicine course, once during my internal medicine clerkship, and once as an intern during a required clinical evaluation exercise. This lack of observation, in hindsight, promoted insecurity about my history taking, physical exam, and patient counseling skills. I had minimal external validation of my competence and little feedback about areas necessitating improvement.

I first became acquainted with Eric Holmboe's work when reading his *Annals of Internal Medicine* article describing how rater training could improve the accuracy of faculty's assessment of residents' clinical skills. At the time, I was overseeing the internal medicine residency outpatient continuity practice at my institution. We invited Eric to our institution to facilitate a workshop designed to train our general internal medicine outpatient faculty in direct observation of residents' clinical skills. My "aha moments" were numerous.

First, observation did not necessitate 30 minutes in the room with a trainee. Frequent brief snapshots were equally valuable, making direct observation feasible and easily embedded into existing work. Second, there were observation techniques that could minimize the intrusiveness of my presence on the resident-patient relationship. Who knew? Third, I learned that accurate assessment requires "breaking down" a clinical skill into its component parts (known as performance dimension training). This task was not easy, and I remember the discomfort I felt realizing that it took thought to identify the knowledge, skills, and attitudes required for a particular clinical skill. Just because we have been trained to be doctors doesn't mean we have been trained to be evaluators. I even experienced a sense of guilt that the performance dimension training got me to think about, in a much more deliberate and concrete way, the important clinical skills I would want to emphasize in my own encounters with patients. It was humbling to admit that I had not really thought about the process of communication since medical school and that many skill areas (such as informed decision making and giving bad news) were not ones I have been explicitly taught. I saw that rater training could be a unique opportunity not only to improve my assessment skills of residents but also to enhance my own clinical skills with my patients.

Fourth, I witnessed firsthand the poor inter-rater reliability of clinical skills performance assessment. Our faculty watched the same exact video trigger tape of a standardized resident with a standardized patient. Some of us would rate it unsatisfactory, some of us would rate it satisfactory, and some of us would rate it superior. This variability in faculty ratings piqued my own interest in clinical skills assessment and rater training, which has subsequently led to a collaborative research program with Eric. We have learned that although there are many tools to guide assessments of residents with patients, assessments using these tools continue to be plagued by issues of inaccuracy and poor psychometrics (i.e., inter-rater reliability). We have explored some of the factors that underlie the variability associated with faculty's assessments of residents after observing them with patients.[10,11] Now, we are using these findings to design and study the effectiveness of alternative approaches to faculty development focused on rater training.

A final key principle for all educational leaders is to never design any program or intervention that depends solely on one person for its success, for to do so is to ensure its ultimate failure. The faculty development course is no exception. I was fortunate to entice Dr. Bill Iobst to join the staff at the ABIM 3 years ago. As a residency program director, Bill attended the course twice, once at Yale and again at the ABIM. Bill has since taken over leadership of the course and together we continue to refine and evolve the training activities to meet the educational needs of clinician-educators in the twenty-first century.

Faculty Development as Innovation

William (Bill) Iobst
Prior Internal Medicine Residency Program Director and Designated Institutional Official, Lehigh Valley Hospital and Health Network, Allentown, Pennsylvania

In 2001, I attended the Evaluation of Clinical Competence Faculty Development Course. At the time, I was a newly appointed Internal Medicine Residency Program director at the Lehigh Valley Hospital in Allentown, Pennsylvania, desperate to understand and implement better program-wide assessment and evaluation. My appointment as program director had coincided with the launch of the Accreditation Council for Graduate Medical Education (ACGME) Outcomes Project. Having not really worked with the old standards, I thought implementing a competency-based approach to residency training would be easy. All I would need to do was learn the new system. However, I became acutely aware of just how hard this transition would be when I had to prepare for a program accreditation site visit by the ACGME. I needed help. Like many clinician educators, my success as a teacher had come through adopting those teaching skills I had seen role modeled by faculty I had respected as a trainee. As a new program director, this approach was inadequate. The twice-yearly APDIM national meetings provided wonderful training, but I was a novice, and I needed intensive training. I literally did not know what I did not know. Fortunately, I chanced upon the Evaluation of Clinical Competence Course. I did not realize it at the time, but this course would change my professional career.

The weeklong immersion into state-of-the-art assessment and evaluation methods was eye-opening. I quickly had a toolbox of assessment and evaluation methods and practical implementation suggestions available for my use. I returned to my program energized and ready to implement change. Over the next 4–5 years, I introduced chart stimulated recall as an assessment of diagnostic reasoning and clinical decision making, calibrated faculty in direct observation skills, began a videotape review program in the residency ambulatory clinic, and began assessing the use of evidence-based searches for resident-generated clinical questions. I started a weekly 2-hour faculty development program for key faculty to help them with these changes in the way we performed assessment.

Of these innovations, I was most enthusiastic about the faculty development initiative. As these sessions evolved, topics expanded from traditional faculty development addressing assessment and evaluation of learners to include a faculty-driven agenda of "professional enrichment." Transitioning to "professional enrichment" was vital to the sustainability of the program and resonated with participants by creating a true learning community with a shared culture. In addition to developing common standards and shared mental models for curriculum and assessment, enrichment topics included the exploration of medicine in literature, the history of medicine, development as mindful practitioners, a book club, and even wine and Scotch tasting. To further develop this community, I sent eight other faculty to the weeklong American Board of Internal Medicine (ABIM) assessment course. This initiative began in 2003. It remains active in spite of my departure from the institution over 3 years ago.

These innovations eventually led to my appointment as the director of network-wide faculty development and to the position of designated institutional officer. However, while locally successful, I was becoming increasingly aware of my inability to implement change on a larger level. I also realized I needed to continue my development as an educator. Balancing work and personal life responsibilities made pursuing an advanced degree in education a non-option. However, one viable option was to revisit what had started me on the road as an education innovator. I registered to attend the Evaluation of Clinical Competence Course for a second time. The course had evolved significantly over the 6 years since I first attended, and I found myself fully reengaged as a learner. The new content was clearly stimulating, but to my surprise, revisiting the unchanged materials was equally rewarding. While I had certainly forgotten significant amounts of the course material, I believe my excitement revisiting the course reflected my evolution as an educator. While I was revisiting familiar material, I was doing so from a different perspective.

Shortly after attending the course, I was offered and accepted the position as the director of academic affairs at the ABIM. This represented the perfect next step for my career and was a once-in-a-lifetime opportunity. My experience as a student of the course, as a program director, and as a local graduate medical education innovator had taught me the need for and power in effective faculty development.

The weeklong immersion course is a powerful catalyst for change, but as supported by the literature, it is not a stand-alone intervention. Attending the course must be combined with a personal commitment to innovate and to disseminate what is learned at our home institutions. I now codirect the course I attended twice as a learner and additionally deliver a significant number of ABIM Faculty Development hospital visits. The hospital visit program takes faculty development in assessment to the training programs at their institution to minimize cost and travel for local clinician educators. I have had the unique privilege of facilitating the development of the Internal Medicine Milestones and the competency-based narrative project that will ideally enhance ACGME accreditation and ABIM certification.[12] I have also facilitated the development of a competency-based approach to cardiology fellowship training and lifelong learning. More importantly, I have been given the opportunity to participate in the evolution of competency-based graduate medical education in this country.

Rarely does significant change perturb the status quo. In graduate medical education, the shift to a competency-based paradigm represented such a change. Such change creates opportunity, and I have been lucky enough to be in the right place at the right time to capitalize on that opportunity. While I am not sure I have found my ultimate destination job, my current position is surely pretty close.

Lessons Learned

Bill powerfully highlights one of the key aspects of faculty development: more than anything else it must serve as a catalyst for continued professional growth of clinical and educational competencies for the participants. Over the first 10 years of the course we have made many changes to keep the course itself up to date and relevant, a journey that has helped to deepen our own understanding of assessment and new competencies and concepts. While the course has produced wonderful individual dividends as a natural by-product, we wish to summarize and emphasize some of our key lessons about faculty development.

- Faculty development has to fill a need for the participants. In short, be sure the faculty development program "provides a meaningful solution to a need or problem" for your participants in their local context.
- The knowledge, skills, and attitudes of any faculty development program have to keep up to date. For Bill and me, the relevance and importance of new research in both medical education and fields outside of medicine in assessment, cognitive science, systems science, and performance appraisal science

over the last 20 years is breathtaking. Just as you expect your participants to implement change based on their faculty development experience, so too must you embrace the need for change in faculty development programs. As the Greek philosopher Heraclitus noted thousands of years ago, "the only constant is change."

- The course has to be adaptable enough to help the participants make meaningful changes in the context of their local environment. The narratives of Chris Smith and Bill Iobst vividly highlight this important principle. We learned that you must be careful not to hold on too tightly to your content and how it will be used; remember the primary purpose of faculty development is its catalytic educational effects. You will not produce experts out of a week- or even monthlong course. The goal is to help create a learning trajectory of success for the individual. That means they will have to make adaptations and add relevant material to meet their needs.

- Seek and use feedback on the faculty development. We've learned a great deal by actively listening to our participants, not only to improve the course but also to expand and deepen our own knowledge and skills in assessment.

- Faculty development must engage and activate the participants. Just as competency-based medical education requires an interactive relationship between the teacher and the learner, faculty development initiatives must engage the participant. Create space and forums for conversation and be comfortable letting some conversations go where they will. These conversations can unearth key lessons and challenges that face educators today – never assume you have "figured it all out" as to what the challenges and needs are for your intended audience no matter how long you've been involved with faculty development.

- One-time interventions are never enough. Prepare the participants to continue their learning and skill development once they leave the course. At the conclusion of each weeklong course, we ask participants to identify at least one "commitment to change" they will begin when they return to their home institutions. While we would like to increase the number of these successfully implemented changes, we are pleased to report that our follow-up survey data shows up to 75% of these changes have been either partially or completely implemented.

- Build evaluation and research, if possible, into your faculty development activities. We have much to learn about faculty development. The discipline and rigor of approaching faculty development from a research perspective can be invaluable in your own personal development while ensuring the faculty development is impactful and effective.[9,10]

- Have fun! The faculty development course is one of the most enjoyable activities we both do at the ABIM. Working with other clinician-educators and medical education researchers is inspiring and rejuvenating and has certainly reassured us that the graduate medical education community has what it takes to successfully transition to competency-based training.

Bill Iobst: Recent and Future Directions for the ABIM Assessment Course

As I mentioned earlier, I attended the course in 2002 and 2007. This experience poignantly highlighted the value of keeping course content pertinent and timely.

As the current vice president for academic affairs at ABIM and Faculty Development Course director, I recognize the need to continually update and adapt the course to meet the needs of those in the field. As the course has evolved, we have focused on meeting this standard by actively seeking attendee feedback and by recognizing evolving approaches to assessment and evaluation of competency.

Attendees have clearly asked for a balanced mix of assessment or evaluation theory and examples of successful application of these theories in practice. As a result, more examples of the successful application of assessment and evaluation tools have been incorporated into course content. Change management strategies and the importance of understanding program and institutional culture are now also discussed.

The course has also responded to advances in the field of competency-based assessment and evaluation. The ACGME charge to develop clearly defined competency milestones and the use of common evaluation tools to document trainee's achievement of these milestones are examples. Course workshops now specifically introduce attendees to the internal medicine milestones,[12] milestones-based assessment using entrustable professional activities,[9] and evaluation using developmental narratives describing learners. Content now also highlights the role competency committees can play in the attestation of trainee competence.

Future directions of the course are likely to reflect the ongoing evolution of competency-based assessment and evaluation, especially as this process relates to the evolving ACGME accreditation system. As the ACGME moves into the "next accreditation system" in the United States, we anticipate evolving content to address the faculty development needs required to ensure that programs can meet these evolving standards.

Attendees have highlighted that attending a 1-week course is a luxury. While we have not changed the length of the course, this feedback has helped focus the goals of the other ABIM-sponsored faculty development initiative, the ABIM Hospital Visit Program. Through this program, ABIM staff travel to institutions that sponsor internal medicine residency programs and deliver an intensive

1-day faculty development program. To complement the weeklong course, these visits now provide a core series of workshops that include an introduction to competency-based medical education, direct observation training, and principles of feedback and assessment. The visit program covers key content from the weeklong course with the goal of disseminating a shared approach and language for advancing competency-based training across the graduate medical education community.

Finally, attendees have consistently requested opportunities to keep the course's learning communities engaged after they disburse. While no such opportunities have yet been developed, we are currently considering multiple options including reconvening cohorts of course attendees for advanced training, sponsoring regional follow-up sessions or reunions potentially at the time of national meetings, and even virtual meetings and communication forums.

Final Thoughts

Participating in and providing faculty development is truly a wonderful experience, and we've had the privilege to work with hundreds of motivated, eager clinician-educators over the last 10 years. Our greatest joy is seeing someone from the course report back their excitement in making a meaningful change in their local culture of educational assessment for the benefit of their learners and program. For each of us personally, faculty development has been one of the most rewarding and personally enriching activities of our entire careers. We hope you find the same joy and satisfaction we have in your own faculty development activities.

References

1. Cook M, Irby DM, O'Brien BC. *Educating Physicians: A Call for Reform of Medical School and Residency.* San Francisco, CA: Jossey-Bass; 2010.
2. Frank JR, Snell LS, ten Cate O, *et al.* Competency-based medical education: theory to practice. *Med Teach.* 2010; **32**(8): 638–45.
3. Asch DA, Nicholson S, Srinivas S, *et al.* Evaluating obstetrical residency programs using patient outcomes. *JAMA.* 2009; **302**(12): 1277–83.
4. Lynn LA, Hess BJ, Conforti LN, *et al.* Clinic systems and the quality of care for older adults in residency clinics and in physician practices. *Acad Med.* 2009; **84**(12): 1732–40.
5. Pangaro L. A new vocabulary and other innovations for improving descriptive in-training evaluations. *Acad Med.* 1999; **74**(11): 1203–7.
6. Hauenstein NM. Training raters to increase accuracy of appraisals and the usefulness of feedback. In: Smither JW, editor. *Performance Appraisal: State of the Art in Practice.* San Francisco, CA: Jossey-Bass; 1998. pp. 404–44.

7. Murphy KR, Cleveland JN. *Performance Appraisal: An Organizational Perspective*. Boston, MA: Allyn & Bacon; 1991.

8. Holmboe ES, Hawkins RE, Huot SJ. Effects of training in direct observation of medical residents' clinical competence: a randomized trial. *Ann Intern Med*. 2004; **140**(11): 874–81.

9. Ten Cate O, Scheele F. Competency-based postgraduate training: can we bridge the gap between theory and clinical practice? *Acad Med*. 2007; **82**(6): 542–7.

10. Kogan JR, Hess BJ, Conforti LN, *et al*. What drives faculty ratings of residents' clinical skills? The impact of faculty's own clinical skills. *Acad Med*. 2010; **85**(10 Suppl.): S25–8.

11. Kogan JR, Conforti L, Bernabeo E, *et al*. Opening the black box of postgraduate trainee assessment in the clinical setting via observation: a conceptual model. *Med Educ*. 2011; **45**(10): 1048–60.

12. Green ML, Aagaard EM, Caverzagie KJ, *et al*. Charting the road to competence: developmental milestones for internal medicine residency training. *J Grad Med Educ*. 2009; **1**(1): 5–20.

6

A Quality Improvement Management Model for Curriculum Evaluation and Integration

Thomas R. Viggiano

Background
. . . .

In 1993, as part of a major curriculum revision, Mayo Medical School implemented a 28-week Pathophysiology course in the second year of the curriculum. This new second-year Pathophysiology course and ten existing first-year interdisciplinary basic science courses composed the Organ System Curriculum. I had been asked to chair both the new Pathophysiology course and the Organ System Curriculum. The most important responsibility I had was to integrate nine units of the Pathophysiology course with ten first-year courses. To integrate the curriculum, it was essential that these courses be critically evaluated.

I learned quickly that the curriculum evaluation system used at our medical school was ineffective. Student response rates were persistently low and the faculty regularly questioned the extent to which student feedback was representative of the opinion of the entire class. Comments made by students often were negative and nonconstructive and contained few suggestions for improvement. Criticisms were directed to individual faculty and at times were personal attacks. The faculty thought that the student comments were inappropriate and rarely helpful for improving the educational program. The students perceived the faculty as defensive and unresponsive to their concerns. It was an unpleasant and unproductive standoff.

There were also some systemic problems surrounding curriculum governance. Our evaluation survey instruments focused on evaluating teaching, not learning. Student feedback commented only on individual courses and not about how an individual course fit into the curriculum. Only one student from each class served on the Organ System Curriculum Committee. Thus, students were only marginally involved in curriculum management. The net effect of these circumstances was that the faculty managed the curriculum without good data or significant input from learners; as a result, little improvement occurred. It was in this context that a system was developed for students to apply continuous quality improvement principles to curriculum evaluation and integration within the Organ System Curriculum.

Quality Improvement Theory and Curriculum Evaluation

Continuous quality improvement (also called total quality management) is a team-based management strategy that emphasizes improvement of the processes by which an organization delivers its product or service. According to quality improvement management theory, an organization is a network of processes (or activities). Continuous improvement occurs by (1) identifying the processes by which the organization delivers its product or service, (2) enabling people who work with the processes to understand their work in relation to customer needs, and (3) empowering people through problem-solving teams to implement process improvements. We applied this theory to curriculum management by (1) defining our service as student learning and identifying our course delivery processes, (2) designing a written survey instrument to evaluate the influence of course delivery processes on student learning, and (3) reengineering our curriculum evaluation system to involve students.

Identification of Processes

We defined student learning as the service our school renders. The processes by which we attempt to accomplish student learning are the activities we engage in to deliver a course or curriculum unit. Focus groups of faculty and students helped to identify eight course delivery processes that influenced student learning: (1) schedule, (2) learning objectives, (3) content, (4) learning resources, (5) instructional methods, (6) examinations, (7) faculty (teaching), and (8) integration of the course into the curriculum.

Written Survey Instrument

Focus groups of students and faculty also developed questions to assess the influence of each of the eight course delivery processes on student learning. A written survey instrument was designed with a seven-point Likert response format scale for responses to specific questions about the effectiveness of each course delivery process in facilitating student learning. A space was also provided for comments and suggestions about how to improve the effectiveness of each course delivery process. The survey instrument was reviewed and approved by the students, faculty, curriculum committee, medical school administrative and secretarial staffs, and deans. Students and faculty were informed that the survey instrument could be modified at any time if the consensus was to do so.

Reengineering of Evaluation System

We also reengineered our curriculum evaluation system to involve more students. A schematic comparison of the former curriculum evaluation system and the new evaluation system is shown in Figure 6.1.

Former Evaluation System

In the existing curriculum evaluation system, all students were asked to complete a written course evaluation survey after taking the final examination in each course. The course evaluations surveys differed for each of the existing ten first-year courses. All of the comments from the class were collected and recorded as a comprehensive evaluation that was usually 7–17 pages long. The comprehensive evaluation comments were sent to the involved course chairs, members of the curriculum committee, and deans. The faculty then discussed the comprehensive evaluation data at the curriculum committee meeting. Only one student from each medical class who served as the permanent representative on the curriculum committee attended the meeting. The faculty interpreted the student feedback and decided how to use it to improve the course.

Reengineered Evaluation System

For the new quality improvement curriculum evaluation system, we communicated to students that their active participation was a demonstration of professionalism and was confidently expected. We also trained our students to give respectful and constructive feedback and to specify the exact improvement needed to solve any problem identified. All students were given an opportunity to volunteer for one or more teams or were assigned randomly. The names of students on the evaluation team were announced before each course. All students

Curriculum Evaluation System

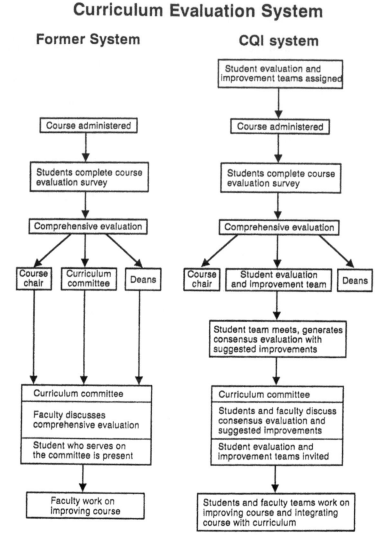

FIGURE 6.1 Reengineering of Curriculum Evaluation System

were encouraged to provide feedback and to suggest improvements throughout the course either by communicating directly with faculty or through the student evaluation team. After the final examination for each course, all students completed the written survey instrument. As previously, the Likert scale responses to the specific questions were tabulated and all comments recorded as the comprehensive evaluation.

The comprehensive evaluation was sent only to the deans, the course chair, and the students on the evaluation team for each course. Within a week after the exam, the student evaluation team met to review the comprehensive evaluation data and formulate a one-page consensus evaluation and set of recommendations.

The consensus evaluation served as an "executive summary" because it prioritized student concerns and made many specific suggestions for improving the course and integrating it with other curriculum units. The consensus evaluation was sent to the involved course chair, the curriculum committee, and the deans, and the consensus evaluation was made available for all students to read. All students on the course evaluation team were invited to the curriculum committee meeting to discuss and clarify the evaluation data.

What Happened: Results

Students, faculty, curriculum committee members, the medical school administrative staff and secretarial staff, and the deans were surveyed, interviewed, or both, to evaluate this new curriculum evaluation system.

After the evaluation system was implemented, the students were very enthusiastic participants in applying quality improvement management principles to the evaluation and integration of the curriculum. Students thought that the course evaluations were being conducted in a more open environment and felt more comfortable expressing their true opinions. The voluntary student response rate increased, the amount of student commentary increased and the comments were more positive, thoughtful, and constructive. There were many specific suggestions for improvement and criticisms directed to the faculty that focused on unproductive behaviors and were stated in a respectful manner. Students thought the consensus evaluation enabled them to speak with "a unified voice instead of making many disparate pleas."

The faculty appreciated the high response rate of the students and accepted the student feedback as representative of class opinion. The faculty agreed that student opinion was more constructive and helpful. At the curriculum committee meeting, the faculty invited the students to elaborate on their suggestions for improving the course and the students perceived the faculty as being more responsive to student opinion. The student evaluation teams volunteered to help faculty implement suggested improvements such as writing clearer course objectives, revising the syllabus, and integrating the course with other curriculum offerings. These faculty-student teams have worked over time to improve the courses, and the students have served as ad hoc curriculum advisers. Even when it was not feasible to implement suggested improvements, the students felt their concerns were being considered.

The curriculum committee believed that the quality of student feedback was more constructive and helpful for evaluating the courses. Faculty and curriculum committee members agreed that the most beneficial feedback from students was addressing curriculum integration. The committee thought that committee meeting time was being used more efficiently and effectively as the committee spent less time trying to evaluate the courses and more time integrating the courses into the curriculum. The committee members also thought that student-faculty communication improved and that the students were more involved in decision making and management of the curriculum.

School administrators thought that student feedback was more helpful, that faculty and student communication improved, and that the new curriculum evaluation system was more effective. The dean agreed that the curriculum evaluation process was more effective and asked other curriculum themes to use this new system.

Observations, Discussion

The idea of applying quality improvement principles to curriculum evaluation and integration was born of necessity. The initial goal of this initiative was to simply generate reliable data that would inform decisions about governing the curriculum. On reflection, I believe this project changed the culture of our school as faculty and students found a way to communicate more effectively and efficiently about our education program and to demonstrate to each other that they both cared deeply about learning. The student evaluation teams continued to work longitudinally to revise objectives, plan schedules, select teaching methods, review examinations and integrate related curriculum content. One of the most satisfying consequences of this work has been to see that students and faculty truly became full partners in managing the curriculum.

The survey instrument was designed to assess the positive or negative influence of curriculum delivery activities on student learning. Analysis of the survey instrument reveals that it assesses the extent to which a learner's four important and interrelated learning tasks were accomplished: (1) student learning was guided by explicit, clearly communicated objectives; (2) learning activities and resources supported the student learning; (3) examinations helped the student assess mastery and deficiency of the desired learning; and (4) the learning experience was coherently integrated with other related learning experiences. The first three tasks are the three essential components of outcome-based education.[1] We have found that student learning is enhanced when curriculum management ensures that these four important tasks are accomplished. Moreover, this evaluation system asks learners to make specific suggestions for improving these important learning tasks.

A very practical benefit of this system is that it generates data that are useful in the medical school accreditation process. The accreditation process for North American medical schools seeks evidence that educational objectives are specified, communicated, and accomplished.[2] Assessing learners' perception of the extent to which a course accomplishes its learning objectives can be used as an outcome indicator of the effectiveness of an individual course. Program level objectives can best be achieved if each course or curriculum unit measures accomplishment of specific objectives and if all courses are integrated into a coherent educational plan. This system also assesses the student's opinion of how different learning experiences are integrated into the curriculum and asks students to suggest ways to enhance curriculum integration.

Jerry W. Swanson, MD, FACP
Professor of Neurology, College of Medicine at Mayo Clinic
Assistant Dean for Assessment and Evaluation, Mayo Medical School

After the implementation of Mayo Medical School's quality improvement curriculum evaluation system, our first 2 years' curriculum was modified. It now consists of blocks of 3 and 6 weeks' duration. The anonymous student surveys are now conducted electronically. At the conclusion of each block, each medical student receives an e-mail reminder to access the integrated scheduling and evaluation system to provide feedback. The electronic form mirrors the original paper form, including questions with Likert scale format responses and the opportunity for each student to provide written, qualitative feedback about changes that he or she would recommend for improvement to the block. All responses are gathered into a summary document, the comprehensive evaluation. The student review team for each block convenes a lunch meeting to review the results.

As assistant dean for assessment and evaluation, I serve as the facilitator and recorder for these student evaluation groups. Each student is expected to participate in an open discussion and contribute to a consensus about how the block delivery processes can be improved. As facilitator, I serve as a guide to assist the review team to come to agreement and prioritize so that recommendations are listed in order of importance. The consensus report is transcribed and sent to each of the five or six student team members with a request for review and comments regarding any suggestions for revision. If any substantive recommendations for revision are submitted, these are communicated to the entire group to be certain that consensus is met. Next, one of the members of the review group sends the draft report to the entire class and solicits feedback. Student feedback is communicated directly to the student review team members to preserve confidentiality. If any recommendations for change in the student consensus report are made, the student review team decides if it is appropriate to change the summary report.

Once this process is complete, the final student consensus report and the comprehensive evaluation from the electronic survey are sent to decanal (dean's) staff, the block chair, and to the curriculum committee. At the curriculum committee meeting, the chair of the block provides her or his overview of the block, discusses the recommendations made in the student consensus report, and outlines a plan for making appropriate changes. Opinions of other members of the committee are sought with an open sharing of ideas as how to best proceed. This includes substantial contributions by other block chairs that may have faced similar issues in their portion of the curriculum. The block chair then works with other faculty members to modify the curriculum for improvement.

Several improvements have been implemented in the curriculum as a result of these cooperative efforts. The faculty members have generally appreciated the candid, respectful feedback of students, and the students have been grateful for the responsiveness and effectiveness with which faculty have addressed the feedback. It has been my observation that students have honestly tried to identify areas that need change and the faculty have made good efforts to implement significant improvements. This has instilled a general attitude of purpose and cooperation in achieving the desired learning, and this has benefited the school. The evaluation process has also helped students to develop leadership skills in teamwork at a relatively early point in their medical education journey. We have observed substantive improvements in the curriculum with subsequent students benefiting from this work. From a practical standpoint, this program helped to provide documentation for a recent Liaison Committee for Medical Education (LCME) self-study and site visit by demonstrating that the curriculum is carefully and effectively reviewed and modified based on student and faculty reflection and efforts.

From a personal standpoint, this work has been very rewarding. The dean recognized my efforts, and he subsequently asked me to chair the LCME Institutional Self-Study Task Force. The efforts of students, faculty members, and support staff led to a successful medical school self-study and LCME reaccreditation visit and to insight into how the school could embrace other opportunities for improvement. By participating in this process, my interest as a medical educator was kindled such that I enrolled in the University of Illinois-Chicago Master of Health Professions Education program. It is my hope that the lessons that I learn in this program will provide me new skills to make additional contributions to Mayo Medical School.

A very meaningful outcome of this work was the opportunity for students to demonstrate "civic professionalism" and to learn by doing. Our students enthusiastically participated in all aspects of curriculum management. At a time when medical educators are challenged to produce future physicians with "new competencies,"[2] our system enabled students to engage actively in learning about teamwork, leadership, evidence-based decision making, systems thinking and quality improvement. When students entered clinical clerkships, they continued to demonstrate problem-solving initiative by troubleshooting problems that were noticed in clinical care delivery processes. We communicated that the "golden rule" for this system was to state the specific remedy or improvement needed for any problem identified. In addition to linking solution generation with problem identification, perhaps the most valuable learning was understanding that if people care enough to make a difference, by working together they usually can.

One of the more powerful motivating forces for this effort was an ironic inconsistency in my daily work. As a physician, I experienced Mayo Clinic's profound commitment to continuously improving clinical services for patients. As an educator, I worked in a preclinical, classroom-based education environment that was much less devoted to improving programs for learners. I believe our students and faculty were not communicating well and regressed into dysfunctional work processes. Each group did not realize how much the other cared about the quality of our educational programs. A positive outcome of this work was that our preclinical environment developed into a student-centered continuous learning system. Another positive outcome was that our students and faculty became the sustaining motivating force for curriculum improvement.

While I was applying quality improvement methodology to my work with the curriculum evaluation system at Mayo Medical School, Dr. John X. Thomas, a friend and colleague, was doing the same at Northwestern University. John and I shared observations and ideas, and discussed strategies that would fit the different contexts and cultures of our respective schools. In our informal collaboration, we sought to achieve similar goals in different medical schools by using quality improvement methodology. John's support, wisdom, and friendship were invaluable to me and I learned from his excellent model of applying quality improvement to curriculum evaluation. Journalist Dale Smith interviewed Dr. Thomas to learn about the experience at Feinberg School of Medicine at Northwestern University. The following is his story.

Moving from Pushback to Professionalism: How Students and Faculty Collaborate on Curriculum Improvement at Northwestern University

Dale Smith
Journalist, University of Missouri, Columbia, Missouri

Throughout the 1990s, the Feinberg School of Medicine at Northwestern University looked passable on paper when it came to using students' input to improve courses and clerkships. The school's curriculum committee included a student along with the 18 faculty members. Each year, the student representative drew from peers' critiques to make suggestions for improving courses and clerkships.

However, in practice this "before" picture of review did little to air students' views and suggestions, says John X. Thomas, senior associate dean for medical education at the school. Student presentations did not incorporate all their peers' reviews, and faculty members often were not receptive to students' ideas.

"The discussions were more like point-counterpoint," Thomas says. "The student would say, 'These exam questions were not worded clearly,' and the course director would respond defensively, 'Well, we do the best we can.'

"Or the student would say, 'Faculty members sometimes contradict one another on points of fact and don't seem to know what the others are teaching,' and the course director would say, 'Faculty members have the right to present their views.'

"As a result, the same complaints arose year after year, and the faculty were not well informed about the issues because the committee didn't communicate well with them. It was an example of well-meaning people struggling within a broken system. Nothing really happened. Nothing changed. Nothing improved."

There was also the problem of asking a lone student to critique curriculum before a committee of faculty members who would likely evaluate the student in another context. Thomas thought there would be strength in numbers by doing it differently. So, he implemented a cyclical improvement process that highlights not only the curriculum's problems but also its strengths. The system offers students opportunities to practice professionalism and leadership while also training them in continuous quality improvement. They use data to design and evaluate the curriculum in a plan-study-act cycle.

The Moving Parts

The new system collects students' ideas more methodically and presents them more compellingly than before. Rather than offering students the opportunity to fill out end-of-course evaluations, the new system requires every student to go online after each exam and anonymously evaluate that segment of the course by answering questions tailored to the purpose. The evaluations are made available to Thomas, course directors, the curriculum committee, and its subcommittee on evaluation.

A panel of students also reviews the evaluations. This group consists of a student senator and up to nine others who volunteer for the year. The panel meets, independently reviews all evaluations, and compiles and prioritizes two or three of the unit's strengths, two or three areas for improvement, and suggestions for course revisions. They distribute this product to course directors and the office of medical education to serve as an agenda for meetings they call.

The Meetings

Review meetings are structured not only to foster amicable and constructive interaction between students and faculty but also to produce concrete ideas to improve courses and clerkships. The groups consist of roughly equal numbers of both groups, including faculty course directors and those who teach the courses. Each student leads part of the meeting, which divides the workload and offers students leadership opportunities.

The presenters offer examples of strength, areas for improvement, and suggestions for changes. Faculty members listen and, if they wish, ask questions or explain their rationale for the topics under consideration. Some ostensibly basic suggestions can lead to substantial changes. For instance, students have pointed out that their premedical education had covered some first-year medical school material. When faculty learned this, they were able to streamline that content.

At other times, the collaborative format leads to conversations and course revisions that would be unlikely to happen any other way, Thomas says. In classes using an audience response to make them more interactive, faculty were at first asking primarily factual questions and occasionally a conceptual question. They were reticent in asking the more abstract questions lest students become frustrated at being asked to deal conceptually with ideas they had not yet mastered. It turns out faculty may have misjudged students' outlook on this matter. "They said the factual questions were not really engaging or interactive," Thomas says. "It was either, 'Yeah, I got it right,' or

'Oh, I got it wrong.' Whereas students found the conceptual questions much more engaging. We heard loud and clear that, even if they got the concept question wrong, it stimulated their curiosity and the realization that they needed to work on it. That is an example of something that happened during the conversation. It didn't leap off the page in the evaluation. But the forum of these meetings allowed such things to come forward."

Thomas adds that a certain social lubricant aided the interaction: "We provide food for these meetings for a very simple reason," he says. "When you're all sitting around eating and drinking and talking, it is more collaborative than confrontational."

After the meeting, students write a short document capturing important discussion points and the resulting action plan. Participants review and approve the document, and students distribute it electronically to their peers, who could see how their comments were used. Each course and clerkship is evaluated every other year, which not only creates a reasonable workload for students but also allows faculty time to revise their offerings and administrators time to manage the process.

From Pushback to Professionalism

Initially, many students suspected that the new process took away some of their independence in critiquing courses and clerkships. Their general perception was that the student panels offered sparse representation. Few understood how the panels were integrated into the larger process of review and revision, Thomas says. Faculty were at first skeptical about whether students would take the process seriously. After all, they'd be offering face-to-face critiques of faculty who may well be evaluating them in courses and clerkships. If students thought faculty would dismiss their ideas, they'd be even less likely to undertake the process in earnest.

The fears of both groups turned out to be unfounded, Thomas says. The us-against-them mentality of the 1990s gave way to more collaborative and professional modes of interaction between faculty and students. "And that's when really good thinking started coming out of this panel process. In one case, several faculty members were told that their materials (PowerPoint, syllabi) weren't as useful as they could be. And the faculty person asked, 'Would any of you be willing to sit down with me and go over this to make sure I understand your perspective?'" In another instance, a student offered up a well-executed diagram from a textbook to replace a hand-drawn illustration the faculty member had been using.

As a result of the new process, faculty now have a better understanding of issues that concern students. "They now have access to constructive information from students that the changes that they are making are helpful. That fuels not only the faculty ego but also the engine that makes the faculty person strive even harder to improve their work."

Students on the review panels also raised expectations for professionalism among their peers. This became clear with regard to students' off-color remarks toward faculty in the evaluations. "We wouldn't edit out nasty comments, partly because we wanted students to participate in a process demanding more constructive course evaluations from their peers. So, there would be instances in which the student senator would get up in front of the class and say, 'We reviewed the student comments, and quite frankly, for a person to make personal attacks doesn't help anything. It is unprofessional, and we are supposed to be striving for professionalism.'"

"Over the years we've seen fewer and fewer unprofessional comments and more of the constructive ones because students knew they were being listened to. So, students know they have a voice and are confident that the faculty are trying to understand their perspective. They begin to see themselves as peers."

Other Outcomes

Internally, the new review system provides a month-by-month longitudinal track record of progress on the curriculum, a record of action regarding feedback and outcomes, and documentation to support faculty development. Externally, it demonstrates to the Liaison Committee for Medical Education that the school has a continuous curriculum evaluation program that includes meaningful student input.

The review system offers concrete evidence of various kinds. If issues that students raised early on no longer arise, then that is considered a sign of progress. It also offers help with difficult decisions. "We have removed some faculty members from key roles because they are impervious to improvement," Thomas says. "It's not about being popular. It's about doing the right things educationally, such as having clear objectives, having access to the best information, writing clear examination questions, being available to answer students' questions, and the like." Students have at times suggested clinical faculty they believed would do well in larger teaching roles. Although the suggestions were at first counterintuitive to administrators, students' instincts turned out to be correct, Thomas says.

The review system provides clear and regular communication from students to faculty members about possibilities for improvement. However, the reverse has been less consistent. "We've asked the unit directors of large courses to devote part of the first lecture to explaining new aspects of the curriculum and to give credit to those who contributed. That's well received when it's done, and I wish I could say that it happens 100 percent of the time. When it doesn't happen, students assume that there have been no changes."

The process fostered a strategic use of resources, especially new technology, Thomas says. As we explored what students brought to the table and what they had seen in other educational environments, it forced us to ask, "Why couldn't we provide this in medical education as well?"

Thomas says that, regardless of shortcomings, the review system is productive, firmly established, and would continue even if key leaders moved on. Both students and faculty value the framework, he says, and so it will remain a fixture at Northwestern.

Reflections on the Experiences of Two Medical Schools

Garvin described a learning organization as "one that is skilled at creating, acquiring, interpreting, transferring and retaining knowledge, and purposefully modifying its behavior to reflect new knowledge and insights."[3] By applying quality improvement principles to curriculum evaluation and integration, both Mayo and Northwestern became learning organizations about education, curriculum, and student involvement.

To our knowledge, the work at Mayo and Northwestern represent some of the first applications of quality improvement in medical education; that is, using improvement concepts and methods to improve the education experience for medical students. Dr. Thomas and I are friends and colleagues. We learned about quality improvement at about the same time. Trading experiences and stories, we supported each other as we sought to apply this new approach to achieve similar goals in two very different medical schools.

Both schools started with a classic feedback-response approach: After each course, the curriculum committee discussed the results, including student feedback. Students were invited to provide written and verbal feedback. The faculty course director was present, but other faculty members involved in the course were not. Changes may or may not have come out of that process. Some of the same student complaints arose year after year.

In the new improvement-oriented systems, teams of students carefully prepared the class feedback and suggestions for improvement. They met with the faculty and worked together collaboratively. Using the "golden rule," students were expected and empowered to contribute to the problem-solving process, not just generate complaints.

There was a strong emphasis on professionalism. Students exerted pressure on their peers to approach the feedback process constructively and with appropriate language.

Over time, the impact was substantial, affecting both the educational activities themselves and also in some cases which faculty members are invited to teach. Students and faculty worked together to improve the flow of learning within and across courses.

As we teach future physicians about the importance of improving care, we believe it is important to role-model improvement in our work as educators. It is important for students to learn that they can make a difference if they work together, use data to analyze problems, communicate effectively, focus on desired outcomes, develop "systems thinking," subordinate self-interests to serve the greater good of their community, and voluntarily exhibit the highest standards of professionalism. In many medical schools, there are limited opportunities to learn these behaviors in the preclinical curriculum. The Mayo and Northwestern models of applying quality improvement to curriculum evaluation improved the learning environment and created opportunities for students to learn these behaviors in a preclinical context. The students continued to exhibit systems thinking and problem-solving behaviors in their clinical years. Thus, the students acquired leadership skills that will help them effectively serve their communities and address the uncertainties of their futures in health care. We hope these models of applying quality improvement to curriculum evaluation are useful to students and faculty at other institutions.

References

1. Shumway JM, Harden RM. Association for Medical Education in Europe Guide No. 25: the assessment of learning outcomes for the competent and reflective physician. *Med Teach*. 2003; **25**(6): 569–84.
2. Greiner AC, Knebel E, editors. *Health Professions Education: A Bridge to Quality*. Washington, DC: National Academies Press; 2003.
3. Garvin DA. *Learning in Action: A Guide to Putting the Learning Organization to Work*. Boston, MA: Harvard Business School Press; 2000.

7

The Dissemination of Relationship-Centered Care Approaches to Enhance the Informal Curriculum of Academic Health Science Centers

*Ann H. Cottingham, Debra K. Litzelman,
Richard M. Frankel, Penelope R. Williamson,
Anthony L. Suchman, and Thomas S. Inui*

Introduction

In 2003 the Indiana University School of Medicine (IUSM) began an experiment, the Relationship-Centered Care Initiative (RCCI), to cultivate the learning environment and professional culture of our academic health center so that it would exemplify the humane values and interpersonal behaviors taught in our formal competency curriculum. Two years later we were delighted to observe real change in faculty and student attitudes, institutional policies, and daily work processes aligned with the project's goals. Knowing that other schools were simultaneously interested in changing their own hidden curricula, we decided to hold a conference that would bring a cadre of schools together to share progress and initiate a learning community around academic health center culture change, the RCCI Immersion Conference. This chapter describes the RCCI and the three RCCI Immersion Conferences that grew out of this activity.

The Relationship-Centered Care Initiative at the Indiana University School of Medicine

Background

The RCCI grew from a fortunate confluence of circumstances. In 2002, Thomas Inui and Richard Frankel joined IUSM. Previously, both served as members of the Pew/Fetzer Task Force on Health Professions Education that had introduced the concept of relationship-centered care. Inui had recently been given funding from the Fetzer Institute to put those concepts into action on an organization-wide scale. IUSM was under the leadership of Dean Craig Brater, who was open to furthering the goals of the initiative. Inui and Frankel assembled a core team working in partnership with the associate dean for medical education and curricular affairs (Deb Litzelman). Like Inui and Frankel, Litzelman had a history of activity in professional development, having been a core member of the IUSM team that created Teaching Caring Attitudes in the late 1990s, a faculty development program designed to improve the ability of the faculty to model and cultivate professional, relational behaviors, and attitudes through their formal and informal interactions with medical students and residents. In 2003, Inui, Frankel, and Litzelman began the RCCI at IUSM. They involved two external

---

Recounting the Birthright Story of the Relationship-Centered Care Initiative

Thomas S. Inui, ScM, MD
Senior Investigator, Regenstrief Institute, Inc.
Indiana University School of Medicine
Director of Research, Indiana University Center for Global Health

I remember difficulty describing to others succinctly what the focus of the Relationship-Centered Care Initiative (RCCI) was going to be at the Indiana University School of Medicine (IUSM). Communicating effectively became especially important as we prepared for the RCCI Immersion Conferences and needed to introduce colleagues at other institutions to our intentions and why they should spend several days "dunking themselves" in our environment.

In our proposal to the Fetzer Institute we had described the RCCI as an experiment in "organizational formation" – assisting or facilitating the IUSM's effort to "respond to a calling" and learn from the experience. At the same time, the RCCI was also intended to embrace a set of activities within which *individuals* on the faculty of medicine at the IUSM would attend to their own personal formation process. "Formation," unfortunately, was a word unfamiliar to academic faculty at the time, except perhaps at Jesuit

---

schools of medicine (e.g., Loyola, Creighton, and Georgetown), where the methods of seminary education were understood. For these reasons the RCCI leadership searched earnestly for a language they could use to communicate the project's intent in a more familiar language to everyone at the IUSM and elsewhere. To this end, we explained that the RCCI was intended to "deepen the expression of professional values" in the organizational environment of the IUSM, relying upon the notion that "professional values" were intrinsic to the concept of medicine as a "calling" and therefore *formation*. This explanation got some traction, but because the word "professionalism" was itself not uniformly understood by faculty, confusion still prevailed.

Finally, with some desperation, I began to say that the RCCI's intent was to (in various ways) help people "take ourselves to work." "Do you remember the typical description of the Old West bar?" I would ask. "The medical school environment is like the obverse of the Old West bar. In the Old West bar, people checked their guns at the door before they went inside. In the academic medical center, we check *ourselves* at the door before we take our *guns* inside. This sad situation has many negative consequences. We should do everything within our power to change it."

Thus, was born the RCCI. We were trying to find ways to take ourselves to work.

---

consultants, Tony Suchman and Penny Williamson, both with extensive experience leading health professional development with the American Academy for Communication in Healthcare. Suchman had recently completed a master's program with Ralph Stacey and was eager to test new theories about human interaction, organizational culture, and culture change in a real-life setting. Williamson had worked closely with Parker Palmer in the development of the Courage to Teach program and brought expertise in facilitating the development of self-awareness and personal formation in multiple venues. This team of Inui, Frankel, Litzelman, Suchman, and Williamson, along with Dave Mossbarger, the program manager, met together over several months and began to develop a plan to achieve a daunting goal: to change the learning environment (informal curriculum) and professional culture of an institution spread over nine campuses and including over 1100 medical students, 1000 residents and 1200 full-time faculty. Other members of the team were added as the program developed, including Ann Cottingham, a colleague with expertise in professional development and communication who had previously worked with Litzelman on the creation of the Teaching Caring Attitudes faculty development program.

Relationship-Centered Care Initiative Strategy

The RCCI was guided by Ralph Stacey's work on human communication and relations called *complex responsive processes of relating*,[1] described in more detail in previous publications.[2–8] Stacey argued that the knowledge, meaning, and patterns of behavior that characterize an organization are constantly co-constructed by the members of the organization in the course of their everyday interactions. Moreover, the formation of these patterns exhibit nonlinear (complexity) dynamics. Previously established patterns may propagate themselves as people enact behavioral patterns in each moment that they think others expect of them. However, new patterns can also emerge, seemingly out of nowhere, as very small new behaviors, deviances from existing patterns, amplify and spread. For example, if a leader decides to invite all the participants at a meeting to share in the creation of the agenda, rather than developing a pre-planned, leader-driven agenda, as might be typical, this new act could influence the attitudes and participation of those attending the meeting. These new attitudes, understandings, and behaviors might then extend beyond that meeting and in turn influence the perceptions and behaviors of others in the organization. These small changes, if they grow and multiply, can have a widespread impact throughout the organization. While potentially powerful, this rippling process of change cannot be predicted or controlled. The leader who chooses to change the practice of agenda-setting at a particular meeting has no way of knowing how this change will impact the meeting participants, nor what each of their responses to the change will be. The outcome of the process set in motion by the leader's small change will depend on the responses of those exposed to the change.

Building on Stacey's theoretical work, the RCCI team recognized that we could not create a detailed blueprint for change because we could not plan or foresee exactly what organizational changes would arise as the process unfolded. Instead, we employed a strategy of *emergent design*. We sought to convene a community of change agents and to foster and support their initiatives. In this way, change tended to emerge spontaneously throughout the project, with each new change influencing others in ways that could not have been pre-engineered or predicted. Instead of creating a full-blown plan, we began with only one planned intervention and observed its results to discern what second step might be possible.

As a first step, the project team consultants (Suchman and Williamson) convened a small group of interested faculty, staff, and students that they called the "Discovery Team" and shared with them the goals and methods of *appreciative inquiry* (AI).[9] The underlying hypothesis of AI is that an organization or individual will tend to move in the direction of its focus, attention, and energy. An organization that attends to what is working well, its areas of strength and success, will motivate additional success, while an organization that focuses on punishment for poor performance and quality by inspection will motivate fear and resentment.

The Discovery Team liked the idea of initiating organizational change through an appreciative process and set out to interview and document the appreciative stories of individuals across the institution. Using a semi-structured instrument, Discovery Team members asked over 80 members of our community to describe times or situations at work in which they had been their very best selves, living their values and being highly effective. Those who were interviewed were invited to interview others, a process similar to "snowball" sampling. The stories collected were disseminated throughout the institution, spreading knowledge of already-existing capacity to achieve the very goals the RCCI hoped to achieve on a larger scale – relationships characterized by authenticity, caring, trust, and respect.

Emerging Interests

As IUSM community members began to think more deeply about their interrelationships and the administrative processes that influenced these relationships, requests for additional training and skills began to emerge. One of the first requests was for training that would help individuals more deeply understand and model what it meant to "be the change they most wished to see in the world," to paraphrase Mahatma Gandhi. In response Suchman and Williamson facilitated a four session, seasonal workshop called the Courage to Lead and invited anyone interested to sign up. Their first cohort filled quickly and the yearlong program was so popular it was repeated and transitioned to Litzelman and Frankel after they completed an intensive 1-year Courage Facilitator training course with Parker Palmer. The Courage to Lead was based on Parker Palmer's well-known Courage to Teach program of personal formation and included the facilitation of self-awareness and abilities to improve capacity to relate effectively with others. To date, 60 of our community have participated in Courage to Lead.

The Courage to Lead program was followed by a request for practical techniques to put relational practices into everyday activities such as meetings and work teams. The Internal Change Agent program was created and led by the RCCI team to meet this expressed need. The program included 28 participants and consisted of five 4-hour sessions focused on the development of knowledge and skills to support organizational change and facilitation. Specific topics included various skills for small-group work, including "checking in," collaboration in agenda setting, communication skills, techniques for understanding and appreciating diverse perspectives, identifying assumptions that could be misleading, and negotiating conflict. The program helped interested IUSM community members become more effective agents of change in our institution.

> I was working in a department that didn't exemplify or embrace the attributes of the RCCI [Relationship-Centered Care Initiative]. While I was doing fine outside the department, the attitude within was abusive and not conducive to a positive learning environment.... Luckily, the RCCI had won over Craig Brater (our Dean) and he was committed to helping us recruit someone (a Chair) who shared in the RCCI values.
>
> —*Jeff Rothenberg, MD, Indiana University School of Medicine*

The IUSM recorded a wide range of institutional developments that evolved from the RCCI between 2003 and 2006. Many are still in place in 2013 and include the following.

- The Admissions Committee developed new competency-based criteria and interviewing methods to select applicants based on values and ability to relate as well as their performance on paper.

- The dean began to include new rigorous data on the work environment in 360-degree performance reviews for department chairs, conducted in a relationship-centered manner.

- A group of students published a book of student stories that was presented to incoming students at the White Coat Ceremony. This project continues and has since expanded and now includes stories from faculty and staff as well.

- The Academic Standards Committee replaced a form letter (known "affectionately" as the "ding letter") with a more relational approach for supporting courses that receive a poor rating from students.

- Practices to "humanize" meetings of the standing committees of the IUSM (e.g., checking in, noticing successes, and appreciative debriefings) were introduced and took hold.

- The School's weekly newsletter, *Scope*, started a relationship-centered column entitled "Mindfulness in Medicine" (a play on "M&M") that focuses on seminal events and experiences of trainees and faculty.

- Techniques such as paired interviewing, reflective narratives, and AI were incorporated into medical education (e.g., chief resident orientation, resident workshops on professionalism, and emerging behavioral and social science initiatives).

All of the changes resulted from self-initiated, voluntary efforts and not from a priori planning. Our dual strategy of AI coupled with emergent design (inviting change to emerge from the interests and actions of interested members of our community rather than mandating a preplanned strategy, as described in more detail earlier) to enhance caring relationships within the larger IUSM organizational environment appeared to be having a significant impact on the relational culture of our organization.

The Relationship-Centered Care Initiative Immersion Conferences

Energized by the positive direction our change process was taking, we decided to share our experiences with other schools of medicine at work on their own organizational and cultural transformations, and reciprocally to learn from those schools about their methods and results. In early 2005, with funding from the Fetzer RCCI grant, we announced our intention to hold a 3-day "RCCI Immersion Conference" at the IUSM that would bring together leadership teams from several other schools where academic medical center cultural change initiatives were under way. Schools were invited to assemble teams of four or five individuals and submit a written proposal describing the culture of their medical school, efforts to transform that culture to date, and the process the team used to complete the application. Teams competed for selection (on the basis of a peer-review of their proposals) and covered their own expenses for travel to the meeting.

Application Process and Attendees

> We chose to come to the conference to enhance professionalism in our faculty and students.
>
> *—Immersion Conference Participant,*
> *University of Wisconsin School of Medicine and Public Health*

Twenty schools applied for participation in the 2005 meeting, nearly one-sixth of all schools in North America. The peer-review process considered the proposed team membership, each school's ongoing cultural change efforts, application quality, and the team process used to develop the application. Eight medical schools were selected as participants for the first conference: Baylor, Geisel School of Medicine at Dartmouth (formerly Dartmouth School of Medicine), Drexel, McMaster, Southern Illinois University, University of Missouri-Columbia, University of North Dakota, and the University of Washington. These schools included private and public institutions, old and relatively new academic medical centers, from the east, west, and central regions of the United States and Canada.

Teams consisted of school of medicine deans, program directors, clerkship and course directors, vice chairs for education, curriculum leaders, student leaders, and other medical educators. The teams gathered in Indianapolis, August 23–26, 2005.

The IUSM went on to host two additional immersion conferences in 2007 and 2008 with residual resources from the Fetzer grant and a second grant from the Arthur Vining Davis Foundations. Participants in these conferences included Columbia, University of Kentucky, University of Minnesota, East Carolina University, Northeastern Ohio Medical University (formerly Northeastern Ohio University College of Medicine), University of Wisconsin, University of Arkansas, University of Nebraska, Harvard, Ohio State University, Ross University, University of California-Davis, University of California–Los Angeles, and University of Virginia. Several schools attended more than one conference and served to bridge ideas and conversations across participant cohorts. At the end of the three events nearly one-fifth of all schools of medicine in the United States had attended at least one of these working conferences.

Conference Overview

> We aspired to create an experience for the participants of being part of a trustworthy, relationship-centered community, while at the same time learning about the RCCI [Relationship-Centered Care Initiative] at IUSM [Indiana University School of Medicine] and sharing culture change enterprises from their own institutions.
>
> —*Penny Williamson, ScD*

All three RCCI Immersion Conferences were filled with intense interaction, new ideas, rich cross-institutional learning, emerging new teamwork, and exuberance. Led by the RCCI team of Thomas Inui, Richard Frankel, Deb Litzelman, Ann Cottingham, and David Mossbarger, along with our RCCI consultants, Tony Suchman and Penny Williamson, the conferences provided an opportunity for schools to discuss their work related to organizational culture and culture change; to explore in depth the concepts of culture, organization, and change; and to sample a range of methods intended to stimulate the development of relational culture.

Enhancing the Professional Culture of Schools of Medicine
IUSM RCCI Immersion Conference III
Program Details

Pre-Conference
Conference planners will participate in a conference call with members from the selected schools to identify "learning edges" to guide program development.

DAY 1 – *Opening Our Eyes, Reclaiming Our Legacy: Acknowledging the Challenges*

8:30 a.m.	Welcome: Deb Litzelman
8:35 a.m.	Professional Cultures of School of Medicine: Tom Inui
9 a.m.	Check-in: Deb Litzelman
9:20 a.m.	Theory of Organizational Change and Relationship-Centered Administration: Tony Suchman
10 a.m.	*Break*
10:10 a.m.	Appreciative Inquiry: Richard Frankel and Dave Mossbarger
10:50 a.m.	Personal Information: Penny Williamson
11:30 a.m.	Plenary Comments and Summary: Deb Litzelman and Richard Frankel
12 p.m.	*Lunch*
1 p.m.	Schools Share Their Stories, "World Café": Penny Williamson
2 p.m.	Open Space Forum: Penny Williamson and Richard Frankel

DAY 2 – *Bringing Fresh Eyes to Work, Discerning the Critical Elements of Our Lifeworld*

8 a.m.	Check-in: Deb Litzelman with Shobha Pais reading poem
8:15 a.m.	Introduction to Organization Fieldwork: Tom Inui and Richard Frankel
9:30 a.m.	Small group preparation – facilitators with each immersion activity group
10:30 a.m.	Travel to immersion activity sites: escorts
11 a.m.	Immersion Experiences, Session A
12:30 p.m.	Immersion Experiences, Session B
2:30 p.m.	Post fieldwork – fieldwork teams
3:30 p.m.	Plenary Reports on Fieldwork Experience: Tom Inui
4 p.m.	Post fieldwork – school teams

DAY 3 – *Finding the Levers for Change at Home: Sharing the Way Forward, Building a National Community of Change Agents*

8 a.m.	Check-in: Ann Cottingham
8:15 a.m.	Personal Formation, Readers' Theater at Tables: Richard Frankel
8:30 a.m.	Planning/Application to Home Institution Challenges: School Teams

FIGURE 7.1 Sample Indiana University School of Medicine Immersion Conference Agenda

I. What is Culture?

> Enhancing the expression of professional values in an organizational environment is – by any other name – altering an organization's culture. The fabric that people within an organization understand to be the web of meanings (e.g., historic origin, contemporary mission, relationship to internal and external stakeholders) that unites them is deeply rooted in values. The difficulty in helping members of any organization recognize these values is that they "live in them" every day. Like "fish trying to think and talk about water," we may not be able to recognize what supports our lives. I hoped to help our Immersion Conference participants "see" and think about the culture in which they swam.
>
> —*Thomas S. Inui, ScM, MD*

What is organizational culture? How can we see and understand the culture of our own institutions? What kind of a culture is best suited for an academic medical center? The Immersion Conference opened with an exploration of institutional culture led by Thomas Inui. He described institutional culture as both a powerful influence on health care trainees and the landscape around us that is difficult to see because it is so familiar. A centerpiece of the RCCI Immersion Conferences was the opportunity for participants to immerse in the IUSM culture. We offered the IUSM as a living laboratory for immersion learning about cultural observation and change, and invited schools to become participant observers and experience our culture in action (the good and the not so good) by attending and taking field notes on a sampling of our ongoing organizational, clinical, educational, and administrative activities.

To prepare for the immersion, Inui led attendees in a participant observation session. Participants viewed a video showing slices of life during a typical day at an academic medical center through the lens of a resident's lifeworld, including rounds, hand-offs, and noon lectures. Immersion Conference participants were asked to identify what these activities revealed about the existing culture of academic medical centers. Passion, dedication to patient care and student learning, and deep knowledge were observed, along with high workload, little time for reflection, hierarchy, and a lack of skilled communication. All institutions represented at the conferences found something familiar in the scenes played out in the clips. After practicing participant observation of institutional culture in the large group, conference attendees set off in small groups to observe and record academic medical center culture in real time using the IUSM as a living laboratory. A wide range of educational, clinical, and administrative activities were offered as fruitful sites for immersion, and each participant selected two for observation. Please *see* Table 7.1 (p. 138) for a sample of the immersion sites and activities.

Following their immersion and observation of the IUSM professional culture and informal curriculum, participants reconvened to debrief their experience. Participants visiting the same immersion site met first to share their responses and observations, then met with colleagues who had observed different sites to share site impressions. Much of what participants observed felt familiar – busy hospital wards, outpatients waiting beyond appointment times, large lecture halls. Some felt different from academic medical center "business as usual." These included activities such as a Council of Elders session, a learning experience during which community elders come together as a panel to share their wisdom about aging and health care with medical students, and a third-year professionalism narrative session, where third-year IUSM students debriefed stories they had written during their medicine rotation that taught them professionalism (good or bad). Novel or familiar, the immersion experiences provided a rich resource for additional thought and discussion about medical school culture.

II. Changing the Culture of an Organization

> We thought of the Immersion Conference itself as an organization. We designed it with the principles of Complex Responsive Process (CRP) in mind and from time to time pointed out what we were doing. In this way, the Immersion Conference truly was a living laboratory, and helped people realize that they already understood the core self-organizing dynamics of CRP: that patterns of thinking and behavior tend to keep themselves going and that very small disturbances in those patterns can sometimes amplify and spread to become transformative new patterns. We introduced such disturbances as new ways of beginning a meeting (check-in), new ways of thinking about change agentry (a curious disturber of patterns rather than an all-knowing designer), and (relatively) new ways of being together (self-disclosure and process reflection). We also created ample opportunity for the teams to initiate disturbances of their own. And it was very gratifying to see the new ways of thinking and the new ways of working together that developed in every team. Some of those new patterns have persisted to this very day. There's no better way to learn something new than to experience it – to be immersed in it!
>
> —*Tony Suchman, MA, MD*

Observations by the teams of outstanding and less-than-perfect examples of professional culture at the IUSM sparked lively discussions of culture change. Any strategy of culture change is founded on some concept of how members of an organization behave and interrelate. Tony Suchman shared with the conference three models of organizational life: the organization as a machine, the organization as an organism, and the organization as conversation. He then explored the implications of these models for planning culture change strategies. Suchman contrasted change strategies appropriate to an organization conceived as a machine, consisting of parts that can be designed (or instructed) to function in a specific way to produce a predetermined product, with an organization conceived as a conversation in which the "product" or end point of a conversation cannot be known at its beginning. A conversation emerges and transforms as each partner shares and responds to ideas in an unpredictable ping-pong of thought.

While a top-down, preplanned intervention might be a logical change strategy if an organization is assumed to function as a machine, an organization understood as a conversation requires a very different approach. From this perspective organizational change is less a matter of identifying a new goal and reprogramming the parts to carry it out than it is a matter of changing the conversation by stimulating new thoughts and interactions among organizational members. Our initial attempt to change conversations by organizing a team to conduct appreciative inquiry interviews caught people's attention. We heard again and again how the interviewers and interviewees enjoyed the opportunity to talk about what had worked well in their work life. It got people across the institution thinking in a new way – with greater mindfulness of the culture they were creating by the way they acted and conversed every day. It also helped to cultivate a group of highly motivated change agents eager to try new relational processes in their normal work activities that might stimulate new thoughts and behaviors in others as well.

One resident story made a lasting impression on everyone. He described a night in the Emergency Department as an internal medicine resident. He was seeing a patient who was going to need admission, and was preparing to call one of his IM [internal medicine] interns who was admitting that night to give him the basics on the patient. This patient was an elderly man being admitted for urosepsis. The resident was conscious of the fact that this kind of admission is not generally eagerly received, so he decided to present the case in a way that might help the intern recognize the true importance of the encounter. When the resident answered his page, he started the conversation by saying, "Hi Andrew. I have a member of the 'greatest generation' who needs your help." It worked.

—Immersion Conference Participant,
University of Virginia School of Medicine

III. Starting with Success

> Appreciative Inquiry (AI) is an organizational change approach that presumes in every organization something is working and that if we ask, How can we get more of what works rather than what's broken and needs fixing, we find ourselves in a different landscape with different perceptions and ideas about what is possible. Bringing together teams from various medical schools to reflect on, and plan changes in the culture of their schools was challenging because of the predominant paradigm in medicine which is one of criticism and negativity. Or, to paraphrase David Leach, past executive director of the Accreditation Council for Graduate Medical Education and an advocate for AI, "if you look for problems you will find more problems." From our work at IU [Indiana University] it was clear that story telling was the best way to demonstrate the power of AI to positively transform the way team members related to one another. Such simple wisdom and guidance in the immersion conferences produced deep, personal and sometimes profound responses in the teams and a model that they could take home and immediately use in their own institutions.
>
> —*Richard Frankel, PhD*

Building on the great success of AI in our own culture change project, we incorporated this method into the Immersion Conferences. Richard Frankel shared the history and goals of AI, and led participants through a round of paired AI interviews. Attendees were asked to reflect on high-point experiences in their own work cultures, times when their work felt most meaningful and in line with their values, when they experienced strong working relationships, and when they had been trusted with responsibility. After a few minutes of private reflection, participants took turns interviewing each other and listening carefully to their partner's stories. Each pair then shared important elements or themes from their interviews with their larger table of eight, and culled themes characterizing meaningful, collaborative work experiences. Similar to the IUSM's experience with AI, all participants were able to identify specific times in their own work experiences when their work and work relationships had been empowering, allowed participants to live their values, characterized by respect, or personally life-giving.

Hands Across the Water, Heads Across the Sky: Immersion and Change across Cultures

Richard Frankel, PhD

Two months after the Immersion Conference, while attending a summer symposium at Dartmouth, I had the opportunity to meet with two members of the Ross University School of Medicine team who had been in Indianapolis, Dean Mary Coleman and Dr. Diana Callender. At that meeting I learned that they were planning to introduce a new competency-based curriculum, and a new Department of Integrated Medical Education that would oversee the new curriculum. Mary and Diana invited me to come to Dominica to do some faculty development using appreciative inquiry (AI) and also consult on how best to introduce Relationship-Centered Care as one of the new competencies.

It was a watershed trip and we were able to introduce the new competency to faculty and staff and do some professional development activities that brought them together around strengths of the school and what it was like at its best. From this meeting an AI discovery team was started. We sponsored a town hall meeting (now known as a "Baraza"*), to hear from students and staff what it was like when they were at their best at Ross.

The Baraza was scheduled toward the end of the day. There was a good deal of concern among the organizers about whether anyone would show up and, if so, what they would say, given the widely held perception that people did not or would not speak spontaneously. As it turned out more than 70 students, faculty, and staff attended. After a brief introduction to AI and describing the goal of the meeting, which was to hear what Ross was like at its best, I invited anyone who had a story to speak.

I remember one story that had a particular impact on me and on everyone who had gathered. A student rose to his feet and explained to the group that he was from Haiti and was on campus January 12, 2010, when the devastating earthquake occurred, and how terrifying it was not to be able to contact family and friends or anyone in the country. With great emotion he described how the Ross community had provided immediate support, organized a relief effort, and made every attempt to help him contact loved ones. He asserted that had it not been for the support he received, he would not have been able to continue as a medical student. Such openhearted sharing brought tears to many in the room as the student expressed his gratitude. The story was transformational and was followed by many more positive stories.

I will carry the memory of what happened that afternoon at Ross with me for the rest of my life. It is one more incredible example of what can happen when people are invited to show up fully and speak from the heart. There is still much work to do, but on that afternoon, I felt incredibly lucky to be invited into the Ross community and privileged to witness the power of the human heart at its best.

Note: *Baraza is a Swahili term that describes a meeting of the community to discuss important matters.

IV. *Be* the Change

In a conversation, the personhood of each conversant, her ideas, behaviors, skills in communication, and personality influence what is said, what is received, and the direction that the conversation will take. The IUSM recognized the importance of personal characteristics for enabling a process of change that is intended to achieve relationship-centered values and behaviors. We therefore included opportunities for personal formation (facilitation of self-awareness and abilities to improve one's capacity to relate effectively with others) and skills development in our own change process as well as in the three Immersion Conferences. During each, Penny Williamson extended an invitation to participants to reflect on a high-point moment in work, a time when "you were your best self, the self you most value and aspire to be." Participants selected a picture from Williamson's vast postcard collection that spoke to them about that time, and then formed groups of three to take turns telling their story and listening to the stories of others in the group. Group members were invited to reflect back to the teller the gifts and strengths revealed in the story and postcard. Whether they had done this exercise one or several times before, all found new, often surprising discoveries about themselves, their personalities, and their capacities. This sample activity demonstrated in a succinct way the power of personal reflection for stimulating the self-knowledge that is foundational for healthy relationships.

> Our intention was for participants to recognize their unique "birthright" strengths and capacities by having peers name them in this activity. Recognizing our own gifts permits us to use them intentionally, to recognize and name them in others, and also to be mindful of our limitations.
>
> —*Penny Williamson, ScD*

V. Humanizing Techniques

> We are a small school, and faculty, staff and students already knew each other, yet we made more of an effort to bring our whole selves to the workplace and to value that in others. We found that our students, rather than wanting "just the facts" were in fact eager for these interactions among themselves and with faculty.
>
> —*Immersion Conference Participant, University of North Dakota School of Medicine and Health Sciences*

We intentionally incorporated into the Immersion Conferences several of the processes that the IUSM adopted to cultivate positive relationships in our culture. These included "checking in," World Café[10] (a process of sharing wisdom through ongoing small group dialogues, described shortly), and Open Space Technology[11] (a process for developing organizational strategy that is participant-driven, described shortly). For example, each morning, participants were seated in small groups at round tables and invited to "check in" with each other before proceeding with the day's activities. The "check in" was an opportunity for each person to share something about him or herself not related to the work at hand, that would help those at the table know them beyond their official role on the team or understand any mental distractions they might be facing that day. It could be a child was playing in an important tennis match that afternoon, or the participant was somewhat distracted by a troubling issue at their home institution, or the participant loved to play the violin and had heard a great concert the night before, and so on. Anything the participant wished to share was

> I remember the surprise of the visiting Deans (participants in the Immersion Conference from other medical schools) who observed an hour-long meeting of the IUSM [Indiana University School of Medicine] Deans. On this particular day the IUSM Deans began their meeting with a 20-minute "check-in," sharing what was top of the mind from their lives and work in order to be fully present to the meeting. They then proceeded to complete the robust work agenda for the meeting in a collaborative and efficient manner. The guests expressed astonishment that so much time would be devoted to seemingly "off agenda" sharing and that these personal disclosures in fact seemed to add to rather than detract from the effectiveness of the session.
>
> —*Penny Williamson, ScD*

invited. Participants were at first highly skeptical about this activity. Concern was expressed that the "check-in" would take up too much of the meeting time, would be uncomfortable, or would come across as "touchy-feely" and off-putting to many. Once they tried it participants were surprised at how quickly this simple introduction took them to a different level of interaction and relationality with individuals they had known for a long time and those they were meeting for the first time. It was a hit at the conferences and a simple technique that attendees could take back to their own institutions.

VI. Sharing Strategies of Change

At each conference, teams were invited to dialogue about their efforts to enhance their own institutional cultures. A modified World Café format was used for this activity. The room was arranged with round tables seating six. Each table of six included one team member from each of six different schools. At least one participant at each table was an alumnus from a previous Immersion Conference (at Immersion Conferences II and III). One member at each table was asked to volunteer to be the table host and remain with the table during the session to welcome participants and share the table's conversation to date with each new round. Team members took turns reporting the work at their home schools and discussing issues related to culture change. At the end of 30 minutes a signal was given for five participants from each table to move to new tables (the host remained), learn from their new host about the conversation to date at those tables, and build on that conversation with reference to the culture change work they were doing at their home institutions. This session included a total of three rounds.

> My colleagues and I went to the first two Relationship-Centered Care Immersion Conferences at Indiana University and came back "on fire," armed to create positive cultural change at Dartmouth...we were better critics of our culture and had tools to be change agents.
>
> *—Immersion Conference Participant,*
> *Geisel School of Medicine at Dartmouth*

VII. An Open Agenda

All of the activities of the Immersion Conferences stimulated reflection, ideas, and questions. An Open Space Forum session was included in the conferences to provide an opportunity for participants to explore areas of interest that had bubbled up throughout the conference in greater depth. True to Open Space, participants created the agenda for the session by developing a marketplace of ideas and self-organizing into groups. Two different time frames were designated so that participants could attend two different sessions or stay for one long session. Participants selected the sessions that they wanted to attend, and were responsible for being fully present in the session and leaving the session to attend another session if their interest lagged or they felt ready to move on. A sample of topics discussed during the Open Space session can be found in Table 7.2.

VIII. Team Plans

We are embarking on a curricular renewal...we will attend to the healing culture, to wellness, support and professional formation, and many of these lessons came from our time immersed at Indiana, the colleagues we met there (a true learning community) and the tools and ideas we returned home with.

—Immersion Conference Participant,
Geisel School of Medicine at Dartmouth

We created Project Professionalism, with goals and plans to enhance professionalism. We set goals to develop our own attributes for professionalism, to start with ourselves in self-examination, and to enhance professionalism in faculty as the best example for students. The goals and plans we developed are still in place and we are closer every year to our goals. We started ways to improve our learning communities, our learning climate, treatment of each other and to encourage dialogue. We integrated narratives in the Medicine and Psychiatry clerkships, discussion sessions regarding struggles in surgery, and went to every department and clinical campus to present on the Optimal Learning Environment and Professionalism, stressing learning by example. We created writers' workshops for our students and faculty.

—Immersion Conference Participant, University of Wisconsin
School of Medicine and Public Health

Throughout the conference, ample time was set aside for colleagues from the same institution to convene as a team and discuss what they were learning from the activities. Each team was asked to collaboratively create a plan to further or initiate a professional cultural transformation process upon returning to their home institutions, and to share their plans with the larger group. On the final

> We began "dropping some stones in the water" as well. One "stone" was to develop a humanism design team composed of basic scientists, clinicians, faculty from philosophy, and first- and second-year medical students. ... The act of bringing together faculty from the basic and clinical sciences and involving both in the planning, implementation, and teaching of these activities did two important things: it opened up discussion of humanism topics from diverse viewpoints and it sent a strong message within the institution – to students, faculty and administration – that these topics are valued among diverse disciplines.
>
> *—Immersion Conference Participant, University of North Dakota*
> *School of Medicine and Health Sciences*

day of the conference each team shared their plans using a World Café format. Each team left with an action plan tailored to that school's individual needs to effect culture change, with ideas such as:

- peer and/or 360-degree evaluations for students, residents, and faculty
- developing or reaffirming an Honor Code
- modifying the admissions and faculty recruiting processes
- modifying the orientation process for students, residents, and faculty
- using appreciative interviews early and often with students
- community meetings
- doing positive storytelling more often
- providing space to reflect, at all levels
- providing positive feedback more often
- including professional attributes and cultural climate in evaluations
- initiate professionalism task forces, websites, and/or portfolios
- establishing consequences for those who don't live the values
- sharing fine arts more, connecting professionally in different ways
- more reward and recognition for those who "go the extra mile" to support peers.

Closing

It is noteworthy that two of the three medical school deans speaking on a panel at a recent Association of American Medical Colleges national meeting on assuring the expression of professionalism in their academic medical center environments cited their participation in the IUSM Immersion Conference as important to their fulfilling the new Liaison Committee on Medical Education accreditation standard regarding the "informal curriculum." As we had hoped, the Immersion Conferences, based as they were, on emergent design and the incorporation of appreciative practices as a cultural norm, spurred new thoughts and creative energy that took root and grew in the organizational DNA of the participating schools.

TABLE 7.1 Sample Immersion Sessions

Activity	Description
Medical Students Shadowing Nurses	The Nurse Shadowing program allows medical students to have an informal lunch with nurses, after which students shadow the nurses for two hours. This experience is designed to foster communication between the two groups and reduce "interprofessional friction." In this session, participants will have lunch with the nurses and discuss the nurses' experiences in this program and with medical students in general.
Interpersonal Dynamics in Root Cause Analysis/Risk Management	Participants will participate in and/or observe a root cause analysis. Participants will observe discussions that will review system issues and avoid blaming language and behavior.
Family as Faculty	Participants will observe the Family-Centered Care portion of Orientation for new or existing staff, during which patient families share their stories related to patient care, and staff ask questions. A Family as Faculty member is someone willing to share the family's story with others in our health care system. That family may or may not have received "family-centered care" and may or may not have uniformly positive things to say. What they share is constructive and intended to help improve care for others.
Patient Safety Interprofessional Grand Rounds	Understanding patient safety from different perspectives of our complex workplace . . . a model of grand rounds to both discuss and model interprofessional education and collaboration.
Narrative-Based Teaching/Learning about Professionalism in Medicine	Participants will observe third-year medical students discussing "professionalism narratives" they have produced during their medicine clerkship. The narratives are de-identified, collated, and given to the students to read during this session. A physician faculty member (Dr. Inui) facilitates group discussion of narratives the students select and assists the students to explore professional themes.
End-of-Life Care Conversations: An Interprofessional Dialogue	Not infrequently the medical care people receive in the hospital seems inappropriate or futile especially toward the end of life. Participants will observe the team of faculty, residents, nurses, and social workers discuss a sentinel event – an unexpected death, a death without named end-of-life care, or an instance of perceived futile care. The goal of these monthly discussions is to provide an opportunity for the various professionals to understand the rational and emotional reasons for the prescribed care and to fully appreciate the impact on the well-being of physicians, nurses, and other staff.
Council of Elders	Participants will observe as students participate in a Council of Elders session during which they interact with a panel of healthy older adults. Students will talk with Council members, discuss how they experience their interactions with the health care system and what would constitute optimal interactions with their physicians.

TABLE 7.2 Sample Open Space Small Group Discussion Topics

How to get involved recruiting culturally sensitive students
How to take the next step to involve the dean with culture change
Engaging chairs and faculty in culture change
Use of narrative to change culture
Breaking down barriers or misunderstanding
Creating a coalition of stakeholders at home around relationship-centered care
Creating cross-organizational networks
Working with residents
How do we conduct a needs assessment of our own informal curriculum culture?
Leadership and change agent development
Starting the uphill climb – empowerment
First steps in changing the culture if there are limited resources
Paradox of planning in an emergent organization

Acknowledgments

The study outlined in this chapter is funded in part by the Fetzer Institute and the Arthur Vining Davis Foundations. This chapter is funded in part by the National Institutes of Health Office of Behavioral and Social Sciences Research and the National Institute of Arthritis and Musculoskeletal and Skin Diseases (Request for Application OD-05-001 – K07).

References

1. Stacey RD. *Strategic Management and Organizational Dynamics.* 3rd ed. Harlow, England: Financial Times Prentice Hall; 2000.
2. Williamson PR, Baldwin DC, Jr., Cottingham AH, *et al.* Transforming the professional culture of a medical school from the inside out. In: Suchman AL, Sluyter DJ, Williamson PR, editors. *Leading Change in Healthcare: Transforming Organizations Using Complexity, Positive Psychology and Relationship-Centered Care.* London: Radcliffe Publishing; 2011. pp. 256–308.
3. Cottingham AH, Suchman AL, Litzelman DK, *et al.* Enhancing the informal curriculum of a medical school: a case study in organizational culture change. *J Gen Int Med.* 2008; **23**(6): 715–22.
4. Inui TS, Cottingham AH, Frankel RM, *et al.* Supporting teaching and learning of professionalism: changing the educational environment and students' "navigational skills." In: Cruess and Cruess, editors. *Teaching Medical Professionalism.* Cambridge: Cambridge University Press; 2008. pp. 108–23.
5. Suchman AL, Williamson PR, Litzelman DK, *et al.* Toward an informal curriculum that teaches professionalism: transforming the social environment of a medical school. *J Gen Intern Med.* 2004; **19**(5 Pt. 2): 501–4.

6. Suchman AL, Williamson PR. Changing the culture of a medical school using appreciative inquiry and an emergent process. *Int J Appreciative Inq Pract*. 2004; May: 22–5.

7. Litzelman DK, Cottingham AH. The new formal competency-based curriculum and informal curriculum at Indiana University School of Medicine: overview and five-year analysis. *Acad Med*. 2007; **82**(4): 410–21.

8. Brater DC. Viewpoint: infusing professionalism into a school of medicine; perspectives from the dean. *Acad Med*. 2007; **82**(11): 1094–7.

9. Cooperrider DL, Srivastva S. Appreciative inquiry in organizational life. *Res Organ Change Dev*. 1987; **1**: 129–69.

10. Brown J, Isaacs D. *The World Café: Shaping Our Futures through Conversations That Matter*. San Francisco, CA: Berrett-Koehler; 2005.

11. Owen H. *Open Space Technology: A User's Guide*. San Francisco, CA: Berrett-Koehler; 2008.

8

Partners in Global Health Medical Education

Learner-Centered Curriculum in Resource-Poor Environments

Paul O. Ayuo, Haroun Mengech,
Robert M. Einterz, and Fran Quigley

THE BIRTH OF MOI UNIVERSITY SCHOOL OF MEDICINE'S CURRICULUM can be attributed to one physician's frustration, but its growth is a result of multinational, multisector collaboration.

Dr. Haroun Mengech, one of the authors of this chapter, joined the University of Nairobi School of Medicine in 1980 as a lecturer in the Department of Psychiatry, a department he later chaired. One of Mengech's most enjoyable experiences in this position was teaching neuroanatomy to first-year students, whom he found to be very inquisitive and highly engaged in their coursework. When Mengech saw those same students in their fifth and sixth years during psychiatry rotations, he noticed they had lost their initiative and seemed to expect only to be told the facts they were to memorize.[1]

In writing and in conversations with his colleagues, Mengech began to question the prevailing medical education process in Kenya, calling for earlier and more intense exposure to clinical training and community-based care. At the same time, the Mackay Commission (1981)[2] on education in Kenya recommended the creation of a second medical school for the country. The new school was to be located in the town of Eldoret in western Kenya, with a curriculum devoted to preventive health care and family health, and with a focus on research relevant to the needs of the community where the school was located. In 1987, Mengech was asked to be the founding dean of the new school, to be called the Moi Faculty of Health Sciences.[3]

Kenya was, and is, a resource-poor environment, with a 40% unemployment rate and half the population living below the poverty line.[4] So Mengech turned to resources outside the country to help him guide the development of the new medical school's curriculum. Supported by a fellowship from the World Health Organization, Mengech visited universities with traditions in the problem-based learning (PBL) model, including McMaster University in Canada, Maastricht University in the Netherlands, and Ben-Gurion University in Israel. Based on his observations and conversations during this tour, and with the collaboration of his new colleagues from around the globe, Mengech began to draft plans to expose all of the new Kenyan school's medical students to community-based clinical education beginning in their first year.

The new school and its curriculum were, and continue to be, grounded in a multinational network of academic health institutions. All of Moi's partners offered assistance in different components of medical education: Maastricht focused its efforts on the PBL foundation of Moi's preclinical medical education, Linköping University in Sweden directed much of its energy to community-based education components, and Ben-Gurion's concentration was on the development of Moi's occupational medicine instruction.[5] As Mengech was preparing to welcome the first class of Moi medical students, a colleague from Nairobi told him, "People from Indiana are looking for a partner, and they are interested in the wild ideas [on curricular reform] you have." Indiana University became the first of several North American schools to partner with Moi in a relationship focused on clinical education and care, along with faculty and student exchange.

At various stages in Moi's development, the partners coordinated through Mengech in an informal "Friends of Moi" consortium and through mutual memberships in The Network, an international group of schools dedicated to community-oriented health education.[6] In addition to expertise, the partner institutions directly provided or helped obtain funding for the new medical school, blunting criticism that a student-based learning curriculum's smaller groups and more labor-intensive approach was too expensive for the government of Kenya.

Concurrently with the development of international networks of support, the new medical school developed multiple layers of connections within Kenya. Before the first class of students ever arrived, Mengech devoted many months to meeting with medical faculty and government officials, building consensus for the new school's innovative curriculum. He interviewed Kenyan physicians in private practice to solicit their ideas for how their medical school training could have better prepared them for the professional challenges they faced. The physicians' suggestions for more student exposure to a wide range of illnesses, better clinical skills training, and guidance on how to manage a health center all found their way into the new school's plans.

A culture of inclusive school management was created, including student input on curriculum and a governance structure with multiple committees. When Moi faculty visited a rural community that was slated to be the site for medical education, care was taken to determine who should lead the community side of the effort. Representatives of the community were invited to sit under a tree where a large circle was drawn in the soil. Mengech or another school official would say, "Tell us who your true leaders are. Put in the circle anyone who you think is critical, anyone you respect. Put in the circle anyone who you will stop and listen to if they are talking." Those so identified by their neighbors became the new medical school's community partners.

By the time the first class of 40 students entered Moi Faculty of Health Sciences in 1990, they were greeted with a curriculum radically different from anything seen in Kenya before. Like the European education system, Moi accepts students immediately out of secondary school into a 6-year medical school curriculum. The first 2 weeks of medical school were devoted to orienting students to what the medical school leaders named the SPICES (Student-centered, Problem-based, Integrated, Community-oriented, Electives and Early clinical exposure, and Systematic) model of innovative medical education. New faculty were encouraged to join in these introductory sessions and learn about their own responsibilities for facilitating self-directed active learning and hands-on health care training. An article describing Moi's innovative learning methods highlighted the value of self-directed learning in a resource-limited environment such as Kenya, citing Kenyan physicians' needs to educate themselves throughout their career in a country where they would have limited access to specialists, continuing medical education courses, professional meetings and corporate-sponsored seminars. In this same article, our Moi University colleague Dr. Peter Nyarang'o praised the value of small group tutorials in preparing medical students to develop skills in managing colleagues and working collegially with other health professionals:

> An additional benefit of group tutorials is that students, through teamwork and individual effort, become competent in group dynamics and communication. Because of the shortage of health professionals in most districts in Kenya, the physician must assume a managerial as well as clinical role. To function effectively as a health team leader, the physician must feel secure and comfortable working in groups.[7]

Students in years one through five were required to spend a minimum of 6 weeks each year in the community, likely in a rural setting. This community-based education and services (COBES) model provided the medical students with exposure to the challenge of seeing beyond the individual patient to grasp community health needs. Students studied the social determinants of health and considered the physician's role in addressing systemic causes of health problems.[8]

Achieving Whatever We Set Our Mind To

Evangeline Njiru, MBChB, MMed
Moi University School of Medicine

I joined Moi University School of Medicine in 1992 and encountered a system of learning that was foreign to me and to most of my fellow classmates. I had no previous experience with problem-based learning, self-directed learning, or certainly community-based education and service, which I only later understood was the effort to make community diagnoses of existing health problems in rural and peri-urban communities.

It took a bit of time to get used to this system, since I had just left high school, where learning was mainly gained through lecturing by teachers. Being involved in the tutorial process initially proved confusing and sometimes bordered on the hilarious. Sometimes all the students had read different textbooks on the same subject, including English, Indian, and British versions, and argued about differing versions of the fundamentals of biochemistry, anatomy, physiology, and other basic sciences. Occasionally, tutors who had no background knowledge of these subjects became confused along with the students!

As time passed by, the process got clearer, students became more accommodating to one another's views, and guidance from the tutors became more enlightening.

Community-based education and services (COBES) was challenging, very interesting, and highly educational. In the initial years of the program in Moi School of Medicine (then known as the Moi Faculty of Health Sciences because it only offered undergraduate training in medicine and surgery), students went for COBES attachment in what we refer to as rural health training centers twice in the first year of medical school and once in the second year. We rotated in different departments in these centers and assisted in weighing children under 5 years of age and pregnant mothers. We also assisted in immunizations, offered clients family planning services, and developed questionnaires for use in the field for community diagnosis.

My first three attachments were at Mosoriot Rural Health Training Centre, and we visited Kapsabet Division and Kosirai Division, both in Nandi District of the Rift Valley Province, Kenya.

We tried to do random sampling in these communities as we applied the questionnaire we had devised. It was grueling work, but I hold fond memories of the hospitality of the people of the Kalenjin tribe in this area, who offered refreshments in every homestead visited. I learned to especially enjoy the famous "mursik," the Kalenjin form of sour milk, often offered in

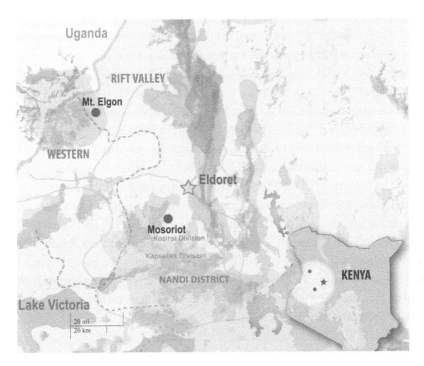

FIGURE 8.1 Rift Valley Rural Medicine Training Sites (reproduced with the permission of AMPATH-Kenya, www.ampathkenya.org)

gourds to our victorious athletes when they returned home from a major championship.

During our third year of medical school, my colleagues and I developed a research proposal that we then implemented in the fourth year. I remember with nostalgia visits to Langas estate of Eldoret town, a slum area where we carried out our research on the burden of worm infestation in children under 5 years of age. On several occasions, household heads declined to have their children provide stool samples because this was taboo in their community. Toiling away in our makeshift laboratory at the university guesthouse, armed with a textbook of parasitology and the assistance of a tutor, we learned how to stain for ova in stool samples and also how to identify ova of different intestinal worms. This self-directed experience proved to my colleagues and I that we could achieve whatever we set our minds to achieve.

COBES in fifth year (COBES 5) was a different ball game altogether. Four of us were posted to Kisii District Hospital, given two rooms to live in, and left to fend for ourselves despite the financial constraints we were in. It was a period during which our teamwork was really tested, including in learning to share household chores. My female colleague Caroline Gichuru and I dug in our heels and refused to be intimidated into doing all the household chores. Our male colleagues had to go to the market too when it was their turn, a thing unheard of in Kisii town then. We were indeed liberated women!

During this 5-week period, our academic responsibilities included rotating in the different clinical and academic departments in the hospital. We interviewed several heads of departments including the medical officer of health, the district public health nurse, and the district public health officer, among others. Unlike other COBES attachments, where the whole group wrote the reports, in COBES 5 every student handed in an individual report.

All in all, COBES had a positive impact on me, helping me to appreciate different cultures, and the community's perceptions of their health problems. What I am today has been influenced by the COBES program: I am more curious, and I look beyond the health problems of a patient to what could be the community-based cause of the illness, what social support the patient has, and what beliefs he has that may influence his adherence to medications prescribed.

Students in Moi's COBES program are trained in the context of the community in which most of them will later practice. Thus, they work with the district health management teams, devise and carry out research projects, and study health promotion and education, epidemiology, biostatistics, disease prevention, and health economics.[9] The COBES model has been demonstrated to effectively enable students to better understand the sources and potential solutions for community-wide health problems, a critically important part of medical education in a country suffering from significant health and poverty challenges.[10] One specific aim of the Moi curriculum is that understanding and appreciation for primary care medicine is inculcated even in medical school graduates who go on to subspecialize.

A Firsthand Glimpse of Health Care Challenges

Jill Helphenstine, MD
Clinical Assistant Professor, Indiana University

I spent the summer of 1998 at Moi University as a first-year medical student. For 6 weeks, two Indiana University School of Medicine classmates and I participated with fellow Kenyan first-year medical students in their community-based education and services (COBES) rotation.

The first-year COBES rotation consisted of 3 weeks of classroom didactic preparation and 3 weeks on-site in a rural community. The 3 weeks of didactic preparation were lecture based and covered topics such as basic epidemiology, basic microbiology, and community entry techniques.

As first-year medical students, our main objective for our clinical "attachment," or assignment, was to conduct an introductory health assessment of a rural sublocation. We were instructed to focus on a relatively small number of homes and interview families regarding their access to health care, their perceived adequacy of health care, and their top health concerns as individuals and a community. During the 3 weeks, we also spent time in the rural health center learning the basic functions of the health center. We gave immunizations and other injections; we drew blood and looked at malaria smears; we weighed babies and plotted growth; we sat with a clinical officer to see patients; and we spent time in medical records and with the pharmacist or pharmacy tech dispensing medicine at the pharmacy.

We also made several visits to different community-based health initiatives. We visited a clean-water initiative based on rainwater collection that was started by a rural women's group, who also did beekeeping to collect and sell honey as a form of income generation for the health initiatives.

The clinical "attachment" piece of the COBES rotation was particularly eye-opening. During our health assessment days, we were divided into small groups. My group consisted of a village elder, a Kenyan classmate who happened to speak the local tribal language, and me. I learned firsthand from local residents about their biggest health concerns: access to clean water and diarrheal disease; access to the local health center (hilly terrain created a nearly 2-hour journey by foot even though the health center was "only" 8 kilometers away); village elders concerned that young girls were leaving school at age 11 or 12 to be married off to older men so that poor families could collect the financially needed dowry; young girls (grade 5 and 6) concerned with how they might protect themselves from getting HIV if forced to marry older men.

After our health assessment was complete, we returned to the sublocation to present a "community feedback" day. Our group of 12 medical students happened to be 50% male and 50% female. We divided the school kids into girls and boys, and the Kenyan first-year female medical students were able to give personal testimony to the value and importance of keeping the young girls in school.

Not only did we learn about local health concerns but also we gained valuable practical skills and spoke firsthand with local people who were involved with locally organized health initiatives. I cannot say enough about the long-term value this COBES experience at Moi University added to my medical education. Through COBES, I gained a firsthand glimpse of the challenges rural Kenyans face in terms of health and access to health care. In my current clinical practice as a pediatrician, I can better recognize the practical barriers to health care that exist for my patients. As a first-year medical student from Plainfield, Indiana, COBES provided a broader perspective, a deeper understanding, and a firmer commitment to global health. With the support of the Gates Foundation funding secured through our partner Indiana University, Moi began work in 2000 to create a postgraduate curriculum. Dean Paul Ayuo, one of the authors of this chapter, spent time at Moi's partner institutions studying their residency programs. He then developed the curriculum for postgraduate programs in Medicine, Child Health and Pediatrics, and Family Medicine. These postgraduate programs lead to a Masters in Medicine (MMed) in addition to providing core clinical training.

What was in 1990 a 40-student Moi Faculty of Health Sciences is now the 650-student-strong Moi University School of Medicine, with 18 departments and 12 postgraduate programs in Nursing (midwifery), General Surgery, Internal Medicine, Family Medicine, Reproductive Health, Medical Education (Master and PhD), Immunology, Child Health and Pediatrics, Radiology and Imaging, Orthopedics and International Health Research Ethics. The school's teaching faculty, once consisting only of Dr. Mengech, now numbers over 100. Growth has not diminished the commitment to student-oriented learning in community settings, and the school now partners with the Kenyan Ministry of Health, both through Moi Teaching and Referral Hospital and the community-based clinics that host COBES training. This multisector collaboration, along with the multinational academic health center partnerships anchored by Moi University School of Medicine, serves as the foundation for the Academic Model Providing Access to Healthcare (AMPATH), one of sub-Saharan Africa's largest and most holistic responses to the challenges of disease and poverty. Founded in 2001 in response to the HIV/AIDS pandemic, AMPATH now treats over 130 000 HIV-positive persons in a clinical network across western Kenya. It includes community-based HIV prevention and a holistic approach to care that provides tuberculosis prevention and treatment, nutrition and income security programs, community-based primary care, and cardiovascular, diabetes, oncology, and mental health treatment.[11]

Maastricht, Linköping, and Ben-Gurion have maintained a steady relationship with Moi as funding and faculty availability allow. Although the North American institutions who are partnering with Moi School of Medicine in AMPATH consciously adopt "leading with care" (or service as a primary focus) as their touchstone, these North American institutions also partner extensively with Moi in research and education, especially in clinical education. In Kenya, faculty from Duke University (cardiology), Brown University's Alpert Medical School (pulmonary medicine), University of Toronto (obstetrics and gynecology), and Indiana University (medicine and pediatrics) help provide clinical training to Moi students. In addition, these institutions and other members of the AMPATH Consortium, including University of Utah, Lehigh Valley Hospital, and Portland Providence Medical Center, host Moi students and faculty for training in their academic health centers.

Physician Problem Solvers

E. Jane Carter, MD
Associate Professor of Medicine, Brown University

I have always viewed the practice of medicine as an opportunity for teaching – whether it was teaching the patient about his disease and how to care for himself or whether it was teaching the student trainees as they rotated through my practice. As a tuberculosis (TB) physician, my focus has also been identification of the barriers that prevent patients from accessing and remaining in care and putting into place programs that address those barriers.

Thus, when I had the chance to travel to Moi in 1997 as a faculty for the medical exchange program, I felt I had identified the perfect spot for me to work and teach. I was especially drawn to the use of problem solving as the basis of the curriculum at Moi, along with a deep appreciation of a public health approach to identification of community health problems through community-based education and services. I also loved the concept of peer-to-peer exchange where my Brown students lived in the dorms with the Moi students and experienced their lives. This concept of peer-to-peer collaborations still remains the basis of the exchange many years later.

These basics were what prompted me, along with my colleagues Dr. Charles Sherman and Dr. James Myers, to approach our dean to formalize Brown Medical School's inclusion in the consortium. Now, almost a decade and a half later, I can look back on several vignettes that demonstrate these core principles, why I think the program endures, and why it succeeds.

Problem-based learning and community-based education and services experiences have shaped the career of many young medical leaders of Kenya who continue to inspire me. For example, following a year as a medical officer in his home district, Dr. Bernard Olayo approached me for advice with the statement, "I know I change lives on a daily basis as a medical officer, but I think with further public health studies I can change more lives through a broader-based approach." He went on to earn a scholarship award to the Harvard School of Public Health, followed by positions as the medical director for the Millennium Village Projects and more recently for the health care team at the World Bank focusing on Uganda, South Sudan, and Kenya. Another example is Dennis Onentia O'yieng'o, who followed his years at Moi with an initiative to begin the first Academic Model Providing Access to Healthcare (AMPATH) affiliated community-based treatment program for multidrug-resistant TB. This program started at a time when the national guidelines emphasized only an inpatient approach. However, Dennis identified the barriers implicit with this approach, designed a safe and effective outpatient program, and piloted it with the blessing of the National TB Program. He presented his work under a travel grant to the American Thoracic Society and now the more comprehensive community-based model for addressing multidrug-resistant TB is the policy of the national program. One final example is Dr. Rose Kosgei. As a medical officer at AMPATH, Dr. Kosgei saw the lack of reproductive care given in conjunction with the HIV care program, where patients had to attend two clinics and stand in two lines to access both reproductive and HIV care. Her design to integrate reproductive care into the HIV care program is now adopted as AMPATH HIV Care policy.

All three of these graduates are products of the Moi University School of Medicine education system. Problem-based learning empowered them to become physician problem solvers, looking at the interactions of individual health problems with systems barriers.

These are only three stories. There are many more. These are the stories that inspire me to be a better physician and a better teacher on a daily basis. I suppose one could say the curriculum at Moi has crafted my approach and teaching style as well. Teachers are supposed to be the inspiration of their students; I have always found it the other way around – particularly at Moi. I believe this is the legacy of the teaching curriculum at Moi.

A less tangible but no less important indicator of success is the acceptance of the problem-based curriculum of Moi University School of Medicine in the Kenyan health professional community. The immediate and obvious competence of Moi graduates has impressed their supervisors and colleagues alike. When one of the school's first graduates went to the traditional University of Nairobi medical school and was voted the best of her class's 100 interns, one of the original skeptics of the new curriculum approached Mengech. "Whatever you are doing, it must be good," he said. "Please continue."

Not a Death Sentence

Fredrick Chite Asirwa, MBChB, MMED, MD
Indiana University, Moi University

My training at Moi University really helped develop my clinical skills, especially my physical exam skills, since students are tasked with so many hands-on experiences from very early on in our education. I found in later experiences with students from more traditional educational programs that I had far more experience than they in physical diagnosis techniques.

I also had a very, very good experience with community-based education and services and found the graduated manner of introducing community health issues ideal. My best experience was in my fifth and final year of community-based education and services, when we conducted a Rapid Rural Appraisal, carrying out a study of the problems we had observed during our third and fourth years in the community.

I was also very fortunate to benefit from Moi University's international partnerships with other medical schools. While still in medical school at Moi, I interacted regularly with visiting students from Indiana University and ended up living with one student's family when I came over to Indiana to continue my education.

I am completing my fellowship in oncology at Indiana University now. My path to choosing oncology was influenced by the care program developed by the Academic Model Providing Access to Healthcare through the partnership between Moi University, Indiana University, and our other international partners. When I was a third-year medical student, every weekend we would wheel 10–12 bodies to the morgue because they had died because of untreated HIV/AIDS. No one would even want to touch HIV patients, and the diagnosis was considered a death sentence. However, through the Academic Model Providing Access to Healthcare, I saw that turn around. Now, I hear people say the same thing with cancer they used to say about HIV: they are told nothing can be done; you need to go home to die.

I want to be a part of providing treatment for early-stage cancer in Kenya, which will not just save those patients' lives but will educate the medical community and the broader community that the disease can be successfully treated if addressed early enough.

There were certainly challenges in implementing Moi's learner-centered curriculum, especially when the school's growth led to more faculty coming aboard with different teaching backgrounds and the larger class sizes forced an increase in the numbers of students in each tutorial group. However, the curriculum continues to be a success. In the authors' opinion, the curriculum is particularly well suited to the Kenyan medical student, who gained admission by performing at the very top of the Kenya Certificate of Secondary Education exam, which determines university admission. The training in PBL, with the main emphasis being problem solving, is especially effective in training an "A" student, who we observe embraces this independent learning style as opposed to being lectured at, which can be tedious for a very bright student. For all students, the skills of debating and reasoning are enhanced through the tutorial process of discussing cases with peers.

Several years after the PBL and COBES programs were fully implemented, Moi faculty interviewed intern supervisors from around the country as part of a curriculum review. The verdict was that intern physicians from Moi stood out compared with those from other institutions in both commitment and reasoned patient management. The immediate former director of medical services also indicated the superiority of Moi graduates in a forum held during the same process. "I can always tell who is a Moi graduate," he said. "A graduate of most institutions will ring and say, 'I have this problem – how do I solve it?' But a Moi graduate will ring and say, 'I had this or that problem and solved it in this or that way. Can I have your approval?'"

In summary, the experience of building an innovative curriculum at Moi University School of Medicine yielded several lessons, including the following.

- Partnerships with academic medical institutions from other countries, especially institutions with experience implementing a PBL model, were critical for curricular development for an institution in a resource-poor environment.
- A culture of inclusive school management and curricular development, including student and community input on design and implementation, reflected the philosophy of PBL and enhanced the development of the curriculum and its embrace by all stakeholders.
- The COBES instruction model provided the medical students with exposure to the challenge of seeing beyond the individual patient to grasp community health needs, especially in the area of primary care.

Acknowledgments

This chapter is funded in part by the Fetzer Institute, the Arthur Vining Davis Foundations, the National Institutes of Health Office of Behavioral and Social Sciences Research, and the National Institute of Arthritis and Musculoskeletal and Skin Diseases (Request for Application OD-05-001 – K07).

References

1. Westberg J. Making a difference: an interview with Dr. Haroun K. Arap Mengech. *Educ Health.* 1999; **12**(1): 108–10.
2. Mackay CB. *Second University in Kenya: Report of the Presidential Working Party.* Nairobi, Republic of Kenya: Government printer; 1981.
3. Quigley F. *Walking Together, Walking Far: How a U.S. and African Medical School Partnership is Winning the Fight Against HIV/AIDS.* Bloomington: Indiana University Press; 2009.
4. Central Intelligence Agency. *The World Factbook: Kenya.* Available at: www.cia.gov/library/publications/the-world-factbook/geos/ke.html (accessed April 4, 2012).
5. Oman K, Khwa-Otsyula B, Majoor G, *et al.* Working collaboratively to support medical education in developing countries: the case of the Friends of Moi University Faculty of Health Sciences. *Educ Health.* 2007; **20**(1): 12.
6. Kaufman A, van Dalen J, Majoor G, *et al.* The network: towards unity for health; 25th anniversary. *Med Educ.* 2004; **38**(12): 1214–17.
7. Nyarang'o P. Kenya's innovation in medical education. *SGIM News.* 1990; **13**(12): 4–5.
8. Odero W. Community-oriented medical education: a strategy for implementing primary health care in Kenya. *SGIM News.* 1991; **14**(5): 4–5.
9. Moi University School of Medicine. Available at: www.chs.mu.ac.ke (accessed March 4, 2013).
10. Pemba SK, Kangethe S. Innovative medical education: sustainability through partnership with health programs. *Educ Health.* 2007; **20**(1): 18.
11. Einterz RM, Kimaiyo S, Mengech HNK, *et al.* Responding to the HIV pandemic: the power of an academic medical partnership. *Acad Med.* 2007; **82**(8): 812–18.

9

An Academic Health Science Center's Journey Toward Teaching and Delivering Patient-Centered Care

Dale Smith

TED GROSHONG'S RÉSUMÉ INCLUDES A DECADE-LONG STINT AS THE University of Missouri (MU) School of Medicine's associate dean for medical education during the time the school overhauled its curriculum – a curriculum that set the stage for its current focus on patient-centered care. But it turns out that his first lesson in patient-centeredness came from the housekeeping staff at a local hospital. Decades later, he continues telling his students this story to show the power of meeting patients on their own terms.

> The summer before going to medical school, I worked as a hospital orderly. One evening, there was a patient who was going to have a gall bladder operation the next day, and she was so worried. The nurse and I kept trying to make her less anxious, but we didn't have any luck. Later, when I went back to change paper towels, a lady from housekeeping was there mopping the floor and talking to the patient.
>
> "Honey, why are you so worried?"
> "Oh, I'm supposed to have surgery tomorrow morning, and I'm so scared."
> "Well, what do you have?"
> "I'm going to have my gall bladder taken out, and I'm just afraid of surgery."
> And she stopped with the mop. "Who's the surgeon that's going to take care of you?"
> "Well, it's Doctor Thomas."

"Ha ha! Honey! You've got nothing to worry about. He's the best surgeon in this place. You've got nothing to worry about. Just relax and get some sleep." And I looked at the patient, and she says, "Wow! That makes me feel a lot better."

So, you've got all these people dealing with this patient, and who did she listen to? The least medically educated person in the entire place. I was very impressed, and I still tell my students about that night.

MU's academic health science center is several years into an initiative that is working to institutionalize patient-centered care as the dominant character-istic of its culture. The approach is comprehensive. For example, the School of Medicine now intentionally enrolls students who have demonstrated abilities and attitudes that indicate they are likely predisposed to deliver patient-centered care, educates them accordingly from their first days on campus, and evaluates their progress. Similarly, the business and clinical operations known as MU Health Care now hire, train, and evaluate employees with patient-centeredness in mind. Finally, leaders across the institution plan health care service lines and construction projects with input from patients. "This initiative isn't just the flavor of the month," says MU Health Care's chief quality officer.

This chapter outlines the journey toward patient-centered care at MU, in terms of leadership, hiring, training, and evaluation; it also includes a focus on students' experiences and infrastructure. The information is drawn from interviews with 14 educational and operations leaders at MU's academic health science center undertaken during 2011. The patient-centered care initiative at MU has many roots, the most important of which appears to be a growing institution-wide ethos among the medical professionals who make up the organization and define its culture.

Those who were interviewed and have the longest institutional memories say there's nothing new about patient-centered care. "I think it's been around forever," said Weldon Webb, associate dean for rural health, "but it used to be practitioner-dependent. When I was young, our small town general practitioner was very patient-centered. The patient was always first, always informed and part of decision-making. The physician knew everything there was to know about the family and managed care accordingly." Webb recalled physicians at MU in the 1970s who were patient-centered, despite infrastructure and sys-tems that worked against it. Several respondents described mentors at MU who taught them patient-centered precepts by word and deed, though such lessons might have been couched in terms of "professionalism" or "doing what's best for the patient."

Critical differences now are that leaders not only articulate a vision for patient-centered care but also provide resources to support it. "It's our culture, it's our mission, it's our values – it's the right thing to do," administrators say.

Singing from the Same Page of Music: How Leaders Foster Patient-Centered Care

Medical education leaders at MU formally articulated the primacy of patient-centered care for the first time almost a decade ago, soon after Linda Headrick, senior associate dean for education, joined the faculty. She recalled, "As a new-comer, I could feel strong institutional values at work with regard to the medical education program, especially the patient case-based, problem-based learning (PBL) aspect of the curriculum, which set the stage for explicitly teaching patient-centered care. I felt that it was important to get these values written down, to reassure everyone that I wanted to preserve and strengthen PBL and to get a consensus to start building from." Faculty accomplished this through the MU 2020 initiative, a planning process that began in 2002. It set out guiding principles for medical education, including foundational values and key charac-teristics that graduates should possess. Here are some of the results of the process that most closely relate to patient-centered care.

Education Mission Statement

> Educate physicians to provide effective patient-centered care for the people of Missouri and beyond.

Foundational Values for Medical Education

> The health of our patients is our first priority. The highest quality health care is the environment for the highest quality education of future physicians.

Key Characteristics of University of Missouri School of Medicine Graduates

The MU 2020 process established eight key characteristics for MU School of Medicine graduates.[1] The first and overarching characteristic is that they be:

> Able to deliver effective patient-centered care: Our graduates are able to deliver care that improves the health of individuals and communities. Effective patient-centered care:

- **Respects** individual perspectives, beliefs, values, and cultures.
- **Shares** timely, complete, accurate, and understandable information to inform health choices.
- **Engages** each person as he/she prefers, understanding that care choices belong to that individual.
- **Partners** in decision-making and the delivery of care.

Our graduates are active participants in the creation of policies, programs and environments that promote care that is patient-centered, grounded in the best available evidence, and conserves limited resources. The care they provide is marked by compassion, empathy, cultural humility, and patient advocacy.

The next step for MU 2020 was to establish educational goals based on the eight key characteristics. More than 100 faculty and students participated in multiple rounds of a Delphi process that produced 15 overall educational goals, or "exit objectives." Several were pertinent to patient-centered care, including interprofessional teamwork. One that stands out is: "Students will demonstrate how to actively engage the patient and pertinent family members and friends in an informed, shared decision-making process while demonstrating respect for their rights, autonomy, and desires."

Many changes in the medical student experience followed, from admissions to curriculum to assessment to student support services to faculty teaching awards. Key elements related to education in patient-centered care are described later in this chapter; *see* "Making the Patient Real: The Medical Student Experience."

One participant in this work asserted that leaders' ability to foster a collaborative spirit among faculty helped advance patient-centered care at MU. "As an innovator, what I need is an environment where I can freely express ideas without being shot down. Innovation stalls at a lot of academic health science centers due to the excessively competitive environment – for tenure, for publications, and so on. That doesn't happen here. I've chosen this place, even though it is 'out in the cow pasture,' because I like the people and thrive in the collaborative environment."

Headrick recalled the excitement of big changes at the medical school during the early years of MU 2020. "But I also had an uncomfortable feeling in the pit of my stomach, since I knew we'd need strong partnerships with clinical leaders. We can't teach patient-centered care if we're not delivering patient-centered care."

The need to more tightly entwine the missions of the medical school and its medical center prompted several actions. For example, Headrick began one-on-one conversations with health system leaders to share the medical education mission and key characteristics and to ask for their help in fostering a patient-centered setting in which students and residents could learn. An MU 2020

Communications Committee formed to find ways of keeping patient-centered goals in the minds of everyone at the academic health science center. The group included a public relations staff member who made numerous contributions including helping to create posters for elevators and PBL rooms.

When Headrick visited high-level hospital administrators, she found they already had taken up the task of shifting the clinical culture toward patient-centered care. Several other respondents agreed that, like at many academic health science centers, MU had plenty of room and plenty of reasons to do better, including improved reimbursement.

"We can see that value-based purchasing is here, and we're going to get paid less if we don't do what everybody thinks we should in terms of caring for patients," said Jim Poehling, assistant vice chancellor for health sciences. He remarked that leaders envisioned a future similar to the 1990s, in which providers were paid a certain amount to manage care for a cohort of people. In that scheme, it's in providers' best interests to keep people healthy and use only necessary resources. "We're trying to anticipate that reform and train physicians to manage it."

Leaders in the health system and School of Medicine launched a quality-focused initiative based on the Malcolm Baldrige framework to improve the focus on patient-centered care. The Baldrige Performance Excellence Program is managed by the National Institute of Standards and Technology, an agency of the US Department of Commerce. The program helps organizations create integrated approaches to performance management. "To change culture requires collective vision and language," one leader said. The framework aims to achieve results by integrating institutional goals with needs assessment, patient preferences, creating a patient-centered workforce, processes and operations. "What ties it together is the measurement and analysis of what we're doing. It's not a program, it's not a fad. It's about fundamentally changing the underlying culture of this organization. It's creating higher awareness of the impact of everything we say, we do, we think in front of our patients – and to think of it from their point of view, rather than our point of view."

In 2008, an MU Health System working group completed the Hospital Assessment Inventory, an evidence-based tool from the Institute for Patient- and Family-Centered Care. Based on the results, the institution developed guiding principles (respect, share, engage, partner); the chief quality officer assembled a Patient- and Family-Centered Care Committee to offer advice on various matters, and set out to develop an infrastructure that supported patient-centered care.

At about the same time, a new position was created that more formally links the medical school with MU clinical operations. The vice chancellor for health affairs oversees both enterprises and reports to the chancellor of the university. One longtime faculty member saw the integration of these three units as a key element in the institution's journey toward patient-centered care. "It is a rare place where the vice chancellor of the system, the hospital CEO and the dean are all singing from the same sheet of music. That is really cool. I've been here 22 years and this is the first time I've seen that. In the past, I've seen a whole lot of electricity at that level and not a lot getting done. If you're not caring about the patient, you're not going to have anything else – research or education – and you're not making any money either. These three have their differences, but it is really cool. It's one of the reasons I took this job [medical director for child health], because I thought we had a really good chance for success."

In 2011, leaders reaffirmed the key characteristics, updated educational goals, and identified three gaps to work on: (1) culturally effective care, (2) population and public health, and (3) professional formation.

Summary

Leaders played key roles in fostering patient-centered care at the school and in the delivery system. They were sensitive to the theme of patient-centered care at the national level and worked to make it part of the local milieu. Leaders from the school and delivery system found each other. Their initiatives, which had begun independently, developed synergy as they collaborated. They codified patient-centered care in initiatives, including MU 2020, quality-improvement activities, and strategic plans. They created a supportive environment in which faculty, staff, and students could learn and practice according to patient-centered goals.

Making the Patient Real: The Medical Student Experience

MU's emphasis on educating patient-centered physicians begins with enrolling students who are predisposed to that approach. For the past few years, the school of medicine has focused its student selection process by working to identify and admit "students who will excel as patient-centered physicians." This process includes reviewing applicants' personal statements for elements that might predict patient-centeredness. Future research will compare those assessments with students' performance on patient-centered examinations (*see* next section, The Curriculum Makes the Patient Real from Day One of Medical Education). This comparison will fine-tune the Admission Committee's ability to select students with the "raw materials" for patient-centered care. The university's medical students have become more service oriented over time, according to the associate dean for graduate medical education.

Before patient-centered care was a topic of widespread interest in the medical profession, an outside assessment of MU's medical education offerings lit a fire at the School of Medicine. School lore has it that in the early 1990s an accreditation team described the university's medical education offerings as "a well-preserved 1960s curriculum." Whether accreditors actually made the remark is in question, but their report did catalyze leaders to shift radically from the school's traditional lecture-based format during the first 2 years of medical school. By 1993, that format had been replaced by what is still occasionally referred to as the "new curriculum."[2] It is a hybrid program built around PBL in small groups, and it includes clinical experiences, coursework on patient care and some lectures. Respondents say the new case-based curriculum not only laid the foundation for teaching patient-centered care to students but it also galvanized the faculty.

"Redesigning the curriculum was a great boost of energy that resulted in tremendous changes and engaged our community of faculty," said one clerkship director. It caused people to work collaboratively around courses and created a sense that, "We can do big things here."

The case-based approach appealed to faculty in both basic sciences and clinical care. The argument to basic-science faculty was that students would learn the basic science better if we put it in the context of the patient. The argument to clinical faculty was that the students would better understand the needs of patients and be more able to contribute in clinical settings. It was patient-centered care without the name.

The Curriculum Makes the Patient Real from Day One of Medical Education

Once students arrive on campus, teaching them patient-centered care requires not only parsing the concept into behavioral objectives and observable behaviors but also providing a climate to support them. "We've done all of those things," said Kimberly Hoffman, associate dean for learning strategies. "We know, through the eyes of our patients and our faculty, what patient-centered care looks like in our institution, and we share those descriptions with students. We've mapped all the places in the curriculum where our students can enhance their ability to deliver patient-centered care." These include standardized patients, clinical experiences, patient-care coursework, assignments asking students to reflect on their progress, and case-based learning scenarios teaching both the basic science and the psychosocial issues embedded in patient-centered care. This approach is built into students' thinking from the beginning. It's part of the fabric, one faculty member commented.

The Legacy Teacher program was created to prompt medical students to reflect on how their interactions with patients influence their professional development. During the third year of medical school, students are invited to submit an essay, poem, or artwork about a patient who has taught them lessons they believe will make them better physicians. Patients and their families are invited to a spring luncheon honoring their contributions to medical education. Third-year students sit with their patients and their families, and a few share their stories from the podium. In 2008, attending the Legacy Teacher luncheon became part of the required second-year curriculum, to set the stage for the patient-centered care expectations of the clinically intensive third year. The event has grown considerably. In each of the past 2 years, one-third of eligible students submitted materials and more than 200 patients, families, students, faculty, and university leaders have attended the luncheon.

Planners have designed multiple evaluations of the curriculum's ability to deliver patient-centered material to students. In addition to successfully completing the tasks mentioned in the previous paragraph, students must pass a new patient-centered Objective Structured Clinical Examination (OSCE) during the third year of medical school.

Faculty developed this challenging exam over more than four years and carefully tested its reliability. It became a requirement for all third-year students in 2011. Kimberly Hoffman observed, "We created complex scenarios that require students to communicate and collaborate with patients, their families and other members of the health care team." These things are assessed during a weeklong evaluation in which students interact with standardized patients during a simulated longitudinal experience. "Perhaps the first time the student meets the patient, is in the hospital with several family members. Maybe they have to get part of the history from a family member. Then we say, 'Now you're coming back six months later and you're seeing the same patient in the ambulatory setting. So the focus of this new OSCE is not only to deliver the care, but to do it in a patient-centered way."

Hoffman also noted that students' strong performances on parts of the OSCE highlight successful teaching, and weaker scores on other segments inform curricular changes. For instance, students did well at breaking bad news to patients. But they were less adept at managing longitudinal relationships. In response, the faculty is working on remedies, which could include recurring paper cases during the first 2 years, continuity clinics during years three and four, or perhaps both.

Fifty faculty members volunteered recently to give 4 hours each to act as evaluators for the OSCE. Preparing to conduct the rigorous evaluations may help this core faculty group solidify a shared understanding of key aspects of patient-centered care.

Making the OSCE a graduation requirement sends students an unmistakable message that they are expected to embrace patient-centered care as their mode of practice. On the other hand, students send messages of their own about patient-centeredness in their clinical environs. For example, students recently began annually completing the C[3] (Communication, Curriculum, and Culture) Instrument.[3] The C[3] Instrument registers students' perceptions of patient-centeredness among clinical role models as well as support for their own patient-centered behaviors and has been used at a number of medical schools in the United States. "We can compare our responses to a cohort group of medical schools, and we look pretty good," Hoffman said.

Students can push a patient-centered agenda in their evaluations of superiors and through their own patient care, according to one residency director. "I just looked at evaluations medical students did in the last 6 months on internal medicine residents, and I think the word patient-centered was in those evaluations three or four times. Students commented, 'This resident was really a nice person and I liked working with him, but he certainly didn't provide very good patient-centered care.' That really shows the culture is different."

The new curriculum's effect is so clear that longtime faculty members sometimes remark upon the improved abilities of third-year students. As evidence, Ted Groshong related the following anecdote. "The curriculum changes not only the way people learn, but the way they practice. We now have third-year students evaluate patients and tell us what's going on physically and psychosocially. Recently, an M3 (student in third year of medical school) on the first week of her clerkship talked about a young patient with high blood pressure. She told me the patient is overweight, but then she says, 'Really, I think the reason she has high blood pressure is that she's being bullied at school.' I asked, Well, why is she being bullied? and the student said, 'She has an odd name and people make fun of it, and she's got braces and glasses. Sometimes they're actually pushing her and other things. And if she has high blood pressure, we know what could happen . . ..'

"So isn't that what you want? Groshong remarked. You don't want somebody who says, 'Her blood pressure is something-or-another, and I think we need to give her a thiazide diuretic.' And before the new curriculum, that's what you would've gotten. This M3 I mentioned knew all about the various blood-pressure medications, but that wasn't the point. She got to the key."

Residency directors at other schools have noticed these qualities, according to several respondents including one residency director. "The medical school here at MU does a really good job of sending patient- and family-centered medical students into residency programs. We have two medical students at Washington University now. And what I've heard from the folks there is that MU students make great residents." Those who are MU graduates are some of the first to go on call because they tend to perform well more quickly, he says. He sees a growing number of young physicians with patient-centered approaches. "If there's a critical mass of people delivering patient-centered care, the light is quickly shined on the people who aren't delivering it."

Summary

Medical school leaders designed a curriculum with patient-centeredness at its heart. The curriculum's cases teach not only basic science but also patient-centered care. Beginning early in the first two years, students have special coursework on patient care, spend time in clinic to observe and practice what they've learned, and complete other assignments that cause them to reflect on this topic. The Patient-Centered Care OSCE, a required evaluation, sends a clear message that they must take seriously the goal of becoming an effective patient-centered physician.

Doing What's Best With the Patient

Michael Bauer, MD
University of Missouri School of Medicine Graduate, Class of 2012

In August 2011, fourth-year medical student Michael Bauer gave a speech reflecting on MU School of Medicine's patient-centered education experience as part of the White Coat Ceremony for the incoming medical school class of 2015. The following is excerpted from those remarks.

I would like to share the story of a man I'll call Mr. Smith, and his family. I'll never forget them. I met Mr. Smith during my first clinical rotation as a third-year medical student at a Family Practice clinic in Springfield, Missouri. My attending physician had been asked to see him at his house. I went along and was so touched by his story that I returned there soon after to sit and talk with him and his family. Mr. Smith was an elderly man who was bedridden due to several chronic medical conditions. The same was true of his wife. He was being cared for by two of his daughters, who rarely left his side. Mr. Smith viewed himself as a man in the traditional sense and as such felt a responsibility to care for his wife and children.

Mr. Smith relied upon his daughters for care, and the daughters had put their lives on hold to care for their ailing parents. He felt he was a burden to them, and he felt guilty that he could not take care of his wife. I spoke at length with Mr. Smith and his daughters about how they handled this situation and how it affected their lives. Upon leaving, he gave me a big smile and thanked me for listening. His daughters were in tears as I left. They hugged me and said they hoped all future physicians would spend time getting to know their patients and families as I had done that day.

After my rotation ended, I found myself calling upon Mr. Smith and his family once again through the Legacy Teachers Program, which honors special patients who have become teachers to medical students by sharing their experiences with us. Part of the program is a luncheon to which we invite patients who had become teachers, to honor and thank them. I contacted Mr. Smith's daughters to invite him to the program only to find out that he and his wife both had died. Their love for each other was so strong that one could not live without the other. They passed away less than 12 hours apart.

His daughters came to the luncheon, where I showed them what the experience had meant to me. It was an emotional time for them as they listened to how their father, though bedridden during the last few months of his life, had had such a strong influence on this medical student. They again thanked me for listening to their father and said he never forgot the day I came over. He frequently had told them how thankful he was to meet a young medical student who brightened his day.

During that rotation, I learned a great deal about what patient-centered care truly means. By discussing with Mr. Smith and his family the nature of his diseases and his prognosis, we, as the medical team, with the support of his family, were able to determine the best care for him in his last months. We could have kept him alive, perhaps for years. But the means required to do so were against his wishes and the wishes of his daughters. We *informed* Mr. Smith of his treatment options, *engaged* him and his family in decision making, *worked together* with him and his family in delivering his care, *respected* his wishes, and were *there for him* and his family emotionally. These five aspects are the cornerstones of delivering high-quality patient-centered care.

And so I say to the Class of 2015 that every patient will become your teacher. You will learn not only about diseases and their management but also how to collaborate with families and colleagues to provide the best quality of care. I admonish you as physicians always to treat patients and their loved ones with the utmost respect and compassion, and never to lose sight of what is truly important in the care of another human being. Each patient is somebody's mother, father, brother or sister, or even friend. Each patient deserves our very best.

I will never forget what my attending in Springfield told me on the first day of the rotation: "It is a *privilege* to see patients. They offer you the deepest and most sensitive aspects of their lives. All patients are to be treated with the utmost respect, as if they were a part of your own family."

The Right People, the Right Training

Although infrastructure, curriculum, and systems all are vectors that help push the academic health science center's culture toward patient-centered care, respondents said that the influence of personnel trumps them all. With patient-centered care as a top priority, the university recently has put in place formal procedures to hire, train and evaluate employees involved in patient care and also support services. This initiative includes interviewing techniques that help select people predisposed to giving patient-centered care, the creation of nearly 80 films of model patient encounters across disciplines, role-playing exercises to teach and demonstrate competence, and formal evaluations by managers. All employees are involved, from the least-skilled staffers to the most sought-after faculty hires.

"We look for a unique kind of individual," said Sue Kopfle, chief human resources officer for MU Health Care. "It's the type of individual who believes in service, who believes that oftentimes when families come into health care, especially hospitals, they're in distress. They understand that, 'This is my community, those are my neighbors, my friends, my family.' We look for the ones who can touch somebody in a time of stress and not just make them well, or make the pain go away. They understand that, 'This is a human being. I want their mind to be at peace at the same time that I'm bringing their body back to a state of health.'"

Hiring

To find such people, a staff of seven recruiters at MU Health Care conducts behavior-based interviews with job applicants. The interview uses a series of open-ended questions in addition to the usual checks on professional qualifications. Some questions pose health care scenarios to which applicants respond by describing how they'd behave. For instance, physicians are asked to imagine themselves describing an upcoming procedure to a patient who looks confused about the conversation. What would they do? "A wrong answer would be, 'Well, if he hasn't asked any questions, then I'd assume everything's fine and I'd just go on.' Or, 'I'd tell my resident to deal with it.' You'd be surprised how many people give those kinds of answers," Kopfle said.

Nonclinical applicants respond to questions about situations they might encounter. Food service workers might be asked how they'd respond if, when delivering food, they noticed a patient was crying. Although they are not expected to engage such a patient, the wrong answer is to do nothing, according to Kopfle. "The right answer is something like, 'I'm going to find a nurse.' You're looking for a person who would never just turn their back and walk away."

Recently, the dean of medicine convinced health system leaders to join him in adding TalentPlus assessment of personality dimensions fitted to the job in question. The scientific talent assessments of TalentPlus are based on the study of successful performance in a given profession or industry, Kopfle says. "The assessments identify candidates with significant potential to succeed in our patient-centered culture. Talent themes including empathy, positivity, relationship-building and outcome-focus are among the desired traits the talent instruments measure. The hospitals and clinics use the assessments for all newly hired or promoted caregivers, and the plan is to incorporate the assessments into hiring for non-caregivers within a year." This new assessment will be evaluated by comparing employees' score with patient satisfaction scores for their units.

Training

After putting in place practices to hire people predisposed to deliver patient-centered care, the next step was training them in the specifics. In 2010, human resources leaders began producing training films to model providers showing respect, engagement, sharing, and partnering. Top employees across disciplines performed in what originally was a set of seven films of encounters that use a local actor who simulated patients in various scenarios during the presentations. Groups of six colleagues watch the 6-minute film, participate in a 1-hour didactic session about patient-centered care and take turns role-playing in various scenarios to practice the behaviors. Group members go to a mock patient room in the clinical simulation center where they act as patients and providers as well as observers who critique the effort. The role-playing is filmed so that participants can compare themselves to the model. Participants also leave with a competencies checklist so they and their managers have a baseline of strengths and weaknesses to work from.

Managers undergo training in how to coach patient-centered care. Back on the units, they observe employees at least monthly and give feedback. "I didn't realize we'd have to do this – we had to teach management how to give honest feedback, and to give it in a way that comes across as coaching. In other words, 'We don't want you to feel demeaned or have your feelings hurt, but we want you to learn,'" Kopfle said.

To date, roughly half of the health system's approximately 5000 employees have undergone the 2-and-a-half-hour training sessions. Although leaders originally were unsure how this initiative would be received, units all over the system have requested their own films.

"At first there was trepidation. People were saying, 'Are you serious, do I really have to go through that?'" Kopfle said. "But they like the role playing, and when they saw their colleagues and their own units in the films, that was a big hit: Now it's, 'Oh my gosh, that's the nurse on 5 East, that's Jamara. I walk down the hall with her every day.' Units are now calling and asking when the patient satisfaction scores are coming out. And they study them. Now you have people wanting the scores to climb, because it's accomplishment, it's achievement."

The satisfaction scores Kopfle referred to are generated from patients' responses to Hospital Consumer Assessment of Healthcare Providers and Systems plus customized questions. Historically, the institution's overall Hospital Consumer Assessment of Healthcare Providers and Systems rank has been as low as the 22nd percentile. However, Kopfle noted that changes in hiring and training have helped lift the scores. "The score is now the 82nd percentile, which means that 74.4 percent of patients give us the top rating of nine or 10."

An example from a medical-surgical floor is emblematic of changes the university hopes will come from its patient-centered care movement. The unit pilot-tested a new shift report, in which incoming and departing nurses were present at the bedside, along with family members if they wished. As nurses shared information with one another, the patient and family were involved, and communication improved, says the director of Patient- and Family-Centered Care. "It's also an opportunity for what we call 'managing up.' The nurse who is leaving might say, 'Mrs. Jones, Chris is going to be your nurse tonight. She's terrific, so you are in good hands.' This way we present information in a way that ensures trust in the relationship. This unit went from the 5th percentile to the 99th percentile in patient satisfaction scores because of changes such as these." Satisfaction scores for physicians on this unit also improved, apparently as a halo effect.

Resident Training

All new residents now take patient-centered care training. The idea is new to many of these physicians, since only about one-third of residents are graduates of MU's medical school with its patient-centered orientation. To help them learn important details, residents study a packet about patient-centered care and are then graded on their performance during a patient-care scenario. They are to demonstrate numerous competencies, including knocking before entering, washing hands, introducing themselves, acknowledging the patient and family, sitting at the bedside, listening for a least 2 minutes without interrupting, and introducing other team members. Although physicians' personal communication styles can remain intact, the exercise is intended to raise the standard for the patient experience.

Fostering the Culture of Patient-Centered Care among Residents

Thomas Selva, MD
Professor of Clinical Child Health, University of Missouri School of Medicine

When new residents arrive each year, Tom Selva, chief medical information officer, *gives a "fire starter" talk as part of their enculturation into patient-centered care. The following text is excerpted from that talk. If he begins in a challenging tone, it's because he wants residents to confront themselves and their ideas about being physicians.*

So, you may ask: What is all this patient-centered care business? Hasn't our whole medical education been about taking care of patients? Isn't that why we went to medical school, sacrificed our youth, and are going deeply into debt? And by the way – who is the patient to tell *me* what to do, what they want, how they want it, when they want it?

  If these sentiments sound familiar, congratulations, you are in touch with the hubris with which the medical profession has practiced its craft

---

for generations. Somewhere along the line, we forgot that we are in a service industry.

If you went to medical school to make money, you'll do OK on that score. But you will miss the emotional and intellectual richness, the wonder, the joy and the tears that make medicine perhaps the most rewarding of careers.

Despite the challenges and frustrations that will fill the days ahead of you, here's what I would say: It's not about you. It's about the patient.

So you may ask again: What is all this fuss about patient-centered care about, and why are we talking about it now? Isn't our niche as doctors to take a history, do a physical, render a diagnosis, and tell the patient what to do? Isn't the patient, ostensibly not anywhere as smart as any of us, supposed to do what they are told? Whatever happened to the sentiment, "Trust me, I'm a doctor"? Doesn't the system move patients reliably along a journey of great care? Short answer: Maybe. There are lots of cracks to fall through. Remember that, in medical care, there's only one person who lives out the entire experience from making the appointment to see their doctor through admission and transition back to their doctor. That's the patient. Indeed, they are the only person who sees all the bills!

Let's think about how we might deal with patients. Let's say the patient is someone you love and respect as you would your own mother. Would you use the same terms with this beloved person as you would with a colleague? Would you start a visit without taking two minutes to look over the chart and get acquainted with her case? Would you open the door without knocking? Would you fail to introduce yourself? Would you wake her up at all hours of the night and then wonder why she looks tired the next day? Would you put her in cold, flimsy gowns that open at the back, call her by a name she doesn't prefer, make her take medicines she doesn't want, and put her on regimens she doesn't understand? Would you refuse to tell her when she can go home or maybe give some nebulous time frame? Would you make assumptions about your beloved patient based on name, nationality, accent, the color of her skin?

Of course not.

Yet, we oftentimes do such things to patients we admit to the hospital or see in the clinic. We dehumanize them, disarm them, "dis-able" them. Occasionally this is appropriate. But even then, do we do so with a clear insight into their humanity and with a clear vision that this is for their benefit? Do we do so with a plan to "re-enable" them – return them to their place in the world?

These issues speak to the core of what we are as physicians. Patients come to us so we can explain their present, predict their future, and change that future.

Patients need our help.

So, go ahead, take it from the top – this time, with some humanity: Take the history by listening without interruption. Do the physical with respect and perhaps some explanation. Order tests with a clear reason. Explain what is wrong. Discuss what will happen should patients choose to forgo therapy or changes in lifestyle. Then work the true art of medicine and change your patients' future by partnering with them to change behavior, alter lifestyle, or start a regimen they can accept, adopt, and sustain.

You are embarking on your residencies. We are committed to teaching you the skills to deliver patient-centered care. It is not "smile school." If you are bored, then you are either (1) not listening or (2) already wired to deliver patient-centered care. But I bet you will gain something valuable from the process.

Let's face it, everybody knows you are smart, the "MD" behind your name speaks to your skills, and we certainly expect that you will do your best to care for your patients. But can you (as they say in show business) *sell it*? Can you communicate that caring? You mustn't assume patients can read your mind and know how much you care. It is about putting yourself in their place.

I promise you that if you place the patient at the core of your professional life, your days will be rich and full and meaningful. To do this, you must put on your game face every day. Take your emotional temperature before entering a room or encountering a family. Use your powerful imagination to walk in their shoes. When we see a patient, we tug on but one thread of the fine tapestry that is their life.

Faculty Training

Similar training – lecture followed by simulated patient encounter – for faculty physicians and residents began in Fall 2011. Before the training, patient satisfaction scores ranked the health system's physicians below average on communication with patients, said Les Hall, then chief medical officer. As of December 2012, almost all residents and faculty (1139) have taken the small group sessions.

Despite pockets of opposition early on, faculty response has been positive. "The medical staff is not a homogeneous lot, by any stretch. We vary in age from just out of training to having practiced 40 or so years," said Kirt Nichols, chief of staff. He says the training will likely be most formative for younger physicians. Reactions to the training have been uniformly positive. When asked to rate the simulation experience on a four-point scale, physicians have on average scored it at 3.93.

Patients appear to be noticing, as well. According to Hall, "As of November 2012, our scores have been above the national average for all hospitals for four of the last six months. This is the first time ever that we have achieved this. And that is, I think, reason for optimism that something we are doing is making a difference."

Summary

Leaders at both the medical school and delivery system agreed that shifting the culture toward patient-centered care requires patient-centered people. Both enterprises now methodically interview prospective employees at all levels of faculty and staff looking for suitable people, and they reject those who they think will not fit in. Next came training. Residents and patient-care staff are now required to undergo simulation exercises to teach patient-centered care precepts, and their superiors evaluate them regularly on these skills. After initial resistance in some quarters, faculty members give the training high marks.

Building Patient-Centered Care into the Bricks and Mortar

Respondents gave examples of how infrastructure could help foster patient-centered care. These ranged from offering patients particular amenities, such as convenient parking, to carefully designing new specialty hospitals that accommodate the needs of providers, patients, and families alike.

Providing single rooms for hospitalized patients is key. Although today's patients and families prefer single rooms, the ramifications for care reach beyond the obvious privacy and space issues that trouble semiprivate rooms.

For example, MU's Pediatrics department recently moved into a building that had been newly reconfigured, a process Ted Groshong had been involved in. It was part of a multiyear effort requesting internal resources to redesign the space with private rooms so that Pediatrics could conduct patient- and family-centered rounds.

"I argued that this is the future of children's care. You don't make rounds in a separate room and then go see the patient, tell him what you're going to do and leave. I think that helped convince the administration. We had unanimous support from the department chairs, too."

"Now I go in with my team to see the patient, and we make decisions with the family there participating, a model I observed at Cincinnati Children's Hospital. We start talking about how the child is doing. Maybe feel like more IV fluids are indicated, and we ask the mother, 'How do you feel about that?' And the mother says, 'You know, I think that's right, I think he's a little dry.' Or the kidney specialist may say to the parents, 'It looks to me like he's a little edematous, but you see him all the time, do you agree?' If so, we say, 'Well then, how about we do some more diuretics to try and get that off.' So, it's really a collaborative effort with the family."

The tour of Cincinnati Children's Hospital also was instructive for another faculty member who was on hand when the question arose of residents' reactions to the more lengthy family-centered rounds. "A resident happened to be bustling down the hallway and spun on her heel, and as she was walking backward down the hallway, said, 'We love it. It saves us two to three hours a day of callbacks from the nurses asking, 'You didn't tell us the plan – the family says this, the orders say that . . ..' At Cincinnati, the patient's nurse is in the room. The medical team writes the orders for the day's plan while in the room, in front of the patient, talking with the patient. That arrangement also helps nurses advocate for their patients."

Conducive infrastructure helps explain why the patient satisfaction score for MU Health Care's Women's and Children's Hospital (WCH) is "sky high" at the 95th percentile, Kopfle said. The university's new Missouri Orthopedics Institute enjoys similar ratings. The facility was built and staffed with patients' moment-by-moment experiences in mind. Parking is available immediately across the street, or patients can exit their cars at the front door and use the valet service. The reception desk is easy to find in the steel-and-glass lobby, and intake rooms for paperwork are only steps away. The facility is aesthetically pleasing, compact and self-contained, Kopfle said. "It's the place where you're going to park, see your physician, have your surgery, recover, eat, go for therapy. You're not trooping thousands of yards to get from one place to another. It's not confusing, it's not big, it's not scary. It was built with patient-centeredness in mind."

Planning for new construction patients will use now includes asking them to critique proposed room designs, one administrator said. "A room may work perfectly for the nurse and the doctor, but if the patient says this room just isn't functional from my point of view, it's a problem. They may say, 'If I'm going to be here, will I be in that chair,' or 'I might want a bottle of water, and you don't have a refrigerator in the room for me.'"

WCH and the Missouri Orthopedic Institute were planned for patient-centeredness partly by soliciting patients' opinions about design. A senior associate dean co-led planning for pediatric services at WCH, including a steering committee of over 40 people that met monthly for 18 months. "The committee included three parents of young patients, whose sole function was to keep us patient-centered," he says. The last item on every agenda was to bring these voices into the conversation. "We'd ask, 'Did you hear anything tonight that makes you nervous? What insights or perspectives can you can offer regarding what we discussed tonight to help us make it more patient-centered. Is there anything we need to be aware of that didn't resonate with you?'" Invariably, the parents offered feedback on topics the committee had forgotten to consider or that never occurred to its professional members in the first place. "They offered perspectives that simply would not have been put on the table had they not been in the room."

Summary

After completing an assessment of patient-centeredness (*see* earlier section, "Singing from the Same Page of Music: How Leaders Foster Patient-Centered Care"), leaders' responses included developing infrastructure that supports patient-centered care. They learned that single rooms are key not only to patient satisfaction but also to patient-centered rounds. Committees that plan construction projects have benefitted from having patients routinely comment on plans.

Conclusion

For more than a decade, MU's academic health science center has worked to develop strategies that institutionalize patient-centered care as its culture's dominant characteristic. The comprehensive approach includes the School of Medicine, which intentionally enrolls students who have demonstrated abilities and attitudes that indicate they are likely predisposed to deliver patient-centered care, educates them accordingly, and evaluates their progress. The initiative reaches into the academic health center's business and clinical operations, which hire, train, and evaluate employees with patient-centeredness in mind. Finally, leaders across the institution plan health care service lines and construction projects with input from patients.

References

1. Headrick LA, Hoffman KG, Brown RM, *et al*. University of Missouri School of Medicine at Columbia. *Acad Med*. 2010; **85**(9 Suppl.): S310–15.
2. Hoffman K, Hosokawa M, Blake R, *et al*. Problem-based learning outcomes: ten years of experience at the University of Missouri-Columbia. *Acad Med*. 2006; **81**(7): 617–25.
3. Haidet P, Kelly PA, Bentley S, *et al*. Not the same everywhere: patient-centered learning environments at nine medical schools. *J Gen Intern Med*. 2006; **21**(5): 405–9.

10

The Power of Doing Meaningful Work Together

Shirley M. Moore

Why Me?

I entered the world of quality improvement education in 1993 with caution and reluctance. I was a new tenure-track assistant professor in a school of nursing in a research-intensive university when my dean asked me to represent the nursing school on a new education project with the medical school. I gently inquired "why me?" She indicated that because I had recently come from a leadership position in a large local hospital, I must know about *quality assurance*. I did have considerable experience with quality assurance, but my goal now was to establish a new identity – that of a researcher and scholar. As I looked around, there were not many tenure-track faculty who were involved in curriculum development projects, particularly those in quality improvement education. (In fact, there was no academic nursing faculty teaching or developing curricula in quality improvement in health care at that time).

I viewed curriculum and teaching projects as the scholarship area of the non-tenure-track faculty, whereas I thought tenure-track faculty did National Institutes of Health (NIH)-funded research. As a new tenure-track assistant professor, I was fearful of being pulled away from my "focus" on research. Staying focused is a strong message given to new tenure-track faculty. When approached by my dean to take on this project (opportunity?) I even had a moment of self-doubt – did my dean ask me to take on this project because she didn't think I had what it took to get research grants? In retrospect, I think that is probably not what she was thinking. I was selected because she knew I had recent firsthand knowledge of quality issues in health care, had experience working across professional boundaries, and generally had good human relations skills to represent the school well in this project. Although I was reluctant and concerned, deep down I knew I was a natural for this project. My fear was that I would like it too much and lose my focus on research. This new project in which I was getting involved was the first national collective of individuals focused on quality improvement education in the health professions – the Interdisciplinary Professional Education Collaborative (IPEC) sponsored by the Institute for Healthcare Improvement (IHI).

My Introduction to a Learning Community

A Local Learning Community

The IHI formed the IPEC in 1994 with assistance from the Health Resources and Services Administration, Bureau of Health Professions, and Pew Health Professions Commission.[1] The aim of IPEC was to equip health professionals with the ability to continually improve the health of the individuals and the communities they served. Cleveland was one of four sites selected to be part of a national collaborative to design and evaluate demonstration projects aimed at integrating continuous improvement in health professions curricula. And we were the first to take on this task. There were no sample curricula, sets of objectives or curricular maps for teaching quality improvement to health professionals in training. In fact, this project was what we jokingly referred to as a "reverse grant" – we received no money, and we paid to participate. Great, I thought. I'm already in trouble with my research trajectory – I'm supposed to bring money into my school, not cost the school money!

It was as part of the IPEC project in 1994 that I met the members of our newly formed Cleveland team – all of whom today are close colleagues in the quality improvement education work that I do and who I credit for the formation of my philosophical approach and passion for the continual improvement of health care. In addition to myself, the initial members of the Cleveland IPEC team were Linda Headrick, MD, associate professor of medicine, Case Western Reserve University (CWRU); Duncan Neuhauser, PhD, professor of epidemiology and biostatistics, CWRU; and Farrokh Alemi, PhD, professor, Program of Health Administration, Cleveland State University. We represented the disciplines of medicine, health management, systems engineering, and nursing. We did not know each other prior to the project and, by training, we had considerably different worldviews. We were brought together by a shared aim, however: to design the first interprofessional quality improvement course for health care professionals in training.

So where does an interprofessional faculty team start when the field they are planning to teach is relatively new and they know little about it, especially when the faculty has not worked together before and hardly know one another? We have described our experiences in more than ten publications (including one in Arabic) and have come to agree that several tasks were important to our success: (1) agreeing on action as a way to accelerate our early learning; (2) reconciling differences in approaches; (3) improving our work together through a series of learning cycles; and (4) developing consensus regarding meeting schedules, work processes, and roles. In other words, as a faculty team, we were committed to being a learning community.

I'm not sure if it was because of the topic – continuous improvement – or if it was the particular set of individuals, or the fact that we were at the leading edge of a movement. Our commitment to one another and to the work at hand has been one of the best work experiences in my career. We felt like pioneers; we were incredibly creative and productive. We watched our students blossom and go on to be leaders in the field of quality improvement. The concept of a learning community was really not used at that time, but I now realize that what we had become as a faculty group was a local learning community. Our philosophy in working together was very simple – do meaningful work together and reflect often. Our faculty team stayed together for 8 years. Many of us still work on projects and publish together despite distance in our places of work. The course we developed, Interprofessional Healthcare Improvement, has been an ongoing vibrant course on the CWRU campus now for 18 years.

National Learning Communities

IPEC was my first deep dive into interprofessional education. It has remained a major focus in my academic career. Most of the education projects in which I have been involved since are because of my promotion of interprofessional collaboration in health care. As part of the IPEC group, I was introduced to two important groups promoting interprofessional work in quality improvement. The first was the IHI. The IHI-sponsored National Forum on Quality Improvement in Health Care is an annual international meeting designed to enhance professionals' learning about the use of continuous quality improvement in health care. Each year at this annual meeting I have been able to maintain my skills and contribute to the growth of quality improvement in health care.

The second important influence on my quality improvement work has been the Health Professional Educators' Summer Symposium. In the initial year of the IPEC project, several leaders of IHI conducted a series of seminars for members of the IPEC groups at a 3-day faculty "training camp" that was held in a country inn in Vermont. The goal of this activity was to teach us the principles of quality improvement and we really needed it. Most of us knew little about quality improvement philosophy and methods. In fact, some of us, like myself, had to shift our thinking from the often punitive, evaluative approaches of quality assurance to the new idea of changing quality through a series of small experiments conducted locally by individuals close to the system in which change was being addressed. We were introduced to the ideas of W. Edwards Deming, Paul Batalden, Don Berwick, Tom Nolan, and others. This initial training camp developed into an annual leadership symposium that has been held each year since 1995. The weeklong gathering brings together an interprofessional community of nurse, physician, and hospital administration faculty committed to leading improvement in health care. My participation in the Health Professional Educators' Summer Symposium since 1995 has been a continual growth and renewal influence on my career.

Interdisciplinary Learning

Geriatric Interdisciplinary Learning Teams

I next became involved in two national demonstration projects that focused on the design and evaluation of interprofessional models of health professions education. In 1996, faculty teams at CWRU in Cleveland, Ohio, and Henry Ford Hospital in Detroit, Michigan, responded to a call from The John A. Hartford Foundation for demonstration projects addressing training for interdisciplinary geriatric health care teams. With additional funding from the Cleveland Foundation, we developed the Learning Team Model, a new model of interdisciplinary training based on the work of Peter Senge.[2] In the Learning Team Model geriatric clinical care teams function as "learning organizations" or "learning teams." These geriatric clinical learning teams are committed to conscious and continuous cycles of learning together. Learners were taught to give and improve care in interdisciplinary teams. Participants were student and practicing nurses, physicians, social workers, and other health professionals. The Learning Team Model was implemented in 22 practice sites across Cleveland and Detroit, including sites providing primary, acute, community-based, and institutional long-term care for older persons. We trained 235 individuals (151 current practitioners and 84 students and residents) in this 3-year project.

Catalyst for Kids

Building on its success in geriatrics, the Learning Team Model was used in another interdisciplinary team training demonstration project involving pediatric primary care settings, the Catalyst for Kids project. Sponsored in 2000 by the Partnerships for Quality Education, an initiative of the Robert Wood Johnson Foundation, Linda Headrick, colleagues from MetroHealth Medical Center, and I began a 4-year project in which medical, nursing, and pharmacy trainees were taught collaborative teamwork skills and continuous quality improvement techniques to deliver and improve the care they give to pediatric patients and their families. Importantly, we showed that the skills of interdisciplinary collaborative teamwork and quality improvement could successfully be taught as part of existing residency and clinical practice training experiences of health professionals.

Why Aren't More Nursing Faculty on Board? A National Nursing Initiative

In the early 2000s, the nurse members of the Health Professional Educators' Summer Symposium began to ask the question of why quality and safety education was not a standard part of nursing education across the country. In fact, it was somewhat embarrassing for us – we were all considered leaders in the quality improvement education field, but we each knew that our own schools of nursing had little in their curricula that addressed continuous quality improvement philosophy or methods. We made a decision that we would lead a nursing initiative to systematically infuse quality and safety into nursing education on a national level and began to seek funding to do this. In 2005 the Quality and Safety Education for Nurses (QSEN) initiative was funded by the Robert Wood Johnson Foundation under the leadership of Linda Cronenwett and Gwen Sherwood at the University of North Carolina at Chapel Hill.[3–5]

As one of the leaders of QSEN, I am amazed at what has been achieved in its short history. Accomplishments include (1) a comprehensive survey of nursing school curricula in the United States to establish baseline data regarding the extent to which faculty teach quality improvement and patient safety; (2) development of education competencies in quality and safety for undergraduate and graduate nursing students; (3) creation and dissemination of faculty development and teaching strategies for the competencies; and (4) completion of pilot projects to test new teaching models of quality and safety in nursing across the country. An annual national conference, the QSEN National Forum, was established and over 400 registrants attended in 2011, only the second year of the meeting's existence. The conference is designed to encourage innovation and assist faculty leaders in the improvement of quality and safety education. We have been aided in our efforts to infuse QSEN competencies into nursing curricula by the American Association of Colleges of Nursing through a series of sponsored training programs focusing on the QSEN competencies for both undergraduate and graduate nursing faculty across the nation.

QSEN leaders also have produced the first comprehensive book on quality and safety education for nurses. Gwen Sherwood and Jane Barnsteiner are the lead authors of the book *Quality and Safety in Nursing: A Competency Approach* to *Improving Outcomes*,[6] which includes a chapter that I contributed on inter-professional education. The QSEN project has been incredibly satisfying – it is now clear that nursing faculty across the country are teaching the requisite knowledge and skills to improve quality and safety in health care. In July of 2012, the QSEN program was moved from the University of North Carolina at Chapel Hill to CWRU to be led by Mary Dolansky, associate professor of nursing. This is a very fulfilling experience for me, as Mary was one of the earliest students in the Interprofessional Quality Improvement Course at CWRU and someone to whom I have been a mentor since her doctoral study years. I look forward to working with Mary as we take QSEN forward on the next level in quality and safety education.

The Veterans Affairs Quality Scholars Program: A National Interprofessional Initiative

An important component of the QSEN initiative was the addition of nurses to the well-established Veterans Affairs National Quality Scholars (VAQS) Program. Established as a physician training program in 1998, the Department of Veterans Affairs Office of Academic Affiliations established the VAQS fellowship at six sites in the country under the leadership of the Dartmouth Institute for Health Policy and Clinical Practice.[7] The purpose of the VAQS fellowship program is to develop health professions leaders with vision, knowledge, and commitment to lead, study, and teach about the improvement of health care in the twenty-first century. It is a 2-year postdoctoral training program that consists of real-world quality improvement projects, a series of videoconferences, national meetings, and other learning activities (e.g., formal education programs and local conferences). Under the guidance of a mentor, the scholars obtain a thorough education in quality improvement, including how to contribute scholarly products to the field.

In 2009, with continued financial assistance from the Robert Wood Johnson Foundation, through QSEN, the VAQS program was expanded to include nurses in doctoral or postdoctoral training. As a QSEN faculty member, I was asked to work with VAQS director, Mark Splaine MD, to codirect this new interprofessional VAQS program. A goal of this intensive training program for the nurse scholars is to produce academic leaders who will develop careers devoted to the advancement of the scholarship of quality and safety. I view the nurses who complete the VAQS program as the first large cohort who will have academic careers that include programs of research focused on quality and safety. These doctorally prepared nurses will lead in advancing the science of quality and safety in health care, and also serve as mentors for the generations of nurse scientists who will follow them.

Building the Science of Quality Improvement in Health Care

• • • • • • • • • • • • • • • •

As a researcher and scholar, I have had a continual drive from my first involvement in the quality improvement movement to promote it as a mainstream academic activity for faculty. To me, this means building and disseminating knowledge in a field – in this case, the field of quality improvement. My belief is that although great strides have been made in teaching health professionals about quality improvement, we have made less progress in advancing the science of quality improvement through research and other forms of scholarship. Fortunately, several health care leadership organizations are now addressing the need to further advance the science of quality improvement. One of the first public forums for sharing new knowledge in the field was the Annual International Scientific Symposium on Improving the Quality and Value of Health Care. This conference was initiated in partnership with the Institute for Healthcare Improvement National Forum and its goal is to encourage, accelerate, and improve the science of continuous improvement in health care and health professions education. This scientific meeting has been an important avenue of dissemination of several of my projects in the field of quality improvement.

Another organization, the Academy of Healthcare Improvement (AHI), was formed in 2005 under the leadership of Linda Headrick, University of Missouri; Mats Brommels, Karolinska University; and Ted Speroff and Robert Dittus, Vanderbilt University. The AHI aims to encourage, advance, and accelerate the science and implementation of continuous improvement in health care and health professions education.[8] The AHI provides strategic direction for the field and offers a set of resources to support individuals across the world who are interested in advancing the field of quality improvement in health care. AHI has been important to me in finding like-minded people who share my desire to advance research in quality improvement.

A Funded Research Project in Quality Improvement

My work in quality improvement remained a "fringe" activity for most of my academic life. It was not until I received tenure in 1998 and was promoted to full professor in 2004 that I felt free to engage more fully in quality improvement scholarly activities. I had a well-established research career that included several NIH-funded clinical trials focusing on cardiovascular risk prevention as well as directing an NIH-funded Center of Excellence in Self-Management Research. I assumed leadership for research development in my school of nursing as an associate dean for research and directed NIH-funded research training grants. With my research career well established, I felt that I could allow myself the luxury of following my passion for improving health care systems. In 2008 when the

Robert Wood Johnson Foundation released a call for grants as part of their initiative to Advance the Science of Quality Improvement Research and Evaluation (ASQUIRE), I saw an opportunity I could not let pass. Colleague Mary Dolansky (as noted earlier, one of my former students in our quality improvement course at CWRU) and I received funding under this initiative to develop and conduct psychometric testing of an instrument to measure *systems thinking*.

Our belief was that knowledge in an emerging field is advanced more rapidly when valid and reliable measures of the concepts central to that field are available. Systems thinking is viewed as a key concept in the success of continuous quality improvement initiatives, yet no valid and reliable instrument existed to measure it. In this project we developed and tested the 20-item Systems Thinking Scale that resulted in an instrument with good reliability and construct and discriminate validity. The Systems Thinking Scale is now publically available for use and information on the measure can be found online at (http://fpb.case.edu/systemsthinking/index.shtm).

At Last, Synergy Between My Research and My Quality Improvement Work

In 2006, I received funding from the NIH for a large trial testing the effect of a new intervention to change health behavior (increased exercise in persons who have had cardiac events). This intervention is based on the use of process improvement methodologies (family or individual use of a series of small experiments to change a daily routine behavior). In collaboration with Farrokh Alemi, who had led our IPEC team in writing a book entitled *The Thinking Person's Guide to Weight Loss*,[9] I designed SystemCHANGE, a novel behavior change intervention that focuses on environmental change using personal system improvement strategies. This trial was a head-to-head evaluation of two different theoretically based behavior change interventions, SystemCHANGE and an intervention based on contemporary cognitive behavioral strategies. The emphasis in SystemCHANGE is on changing systems in people's lives rather than relying on motivation or memory for health behavior change. This trial is now completed and in an award-winning abstract, the findings were recently reported at the American Heart Association Scientific Sessions. Not surprising to us in the field of continuous quality improvement, the SystemCHANGE group had superior outcomes. I am pleased to report that SystemCHANGE is now being tested for its effectiveness to produce health behavior change in several other populations, including persons with HIV or stroke and adolescents struggling with weight management. I am now in the process of creating SystemCHANGE toolkits that health care professionals can use to assist individuals in behavior change processes associated with diet, exercise, weight management, and medication adherence. Indeed, my quality improvement work and research have melded.

A Mentor Like No Other

Mary A. Dolansky, PhD, RN
Assistant Professor of Nursing, Frances Payne Bolton School of Nursing, Case Western Reserve University

"A passion to improve health care," that was the magnet the drew me to Shirley Moore, RN, PhD. Shirley, my career mentor, exudes energy around quality and safety and her ideas and projects are incredibly innovative and different. She has a quality improvement philosophy that provides the foundation for her success in teaching and research. She has taught me to use improvement tools personally and professionally. One of my favorites is the use of cycles of change for scholarly writing – running Plan-Do-Study-Act (PDSA) cycles to meet the goal of writing for 30 minutes a day. I even observe improvement philosophy in her leadership roles at the School of Nursing where she implemented improvement principles to increase the efficiency and quality of grant submissions in the center for research. She is a pioneer, determined to unearth new ways of thinking to promote quality improvement in health care.

So when did this mentor "like no other" come into my life and influence my thinking? I began to work with Shirley as a student research assistant on a pilot study she was conducting. I was intrigued with how she managed the study meetings and used quality improvement tools. At this time, she was teaching a class on the application of improvement principles to help patients make behavior changes. It was a very different approach. I tried the techniques with my family members and watched them go through cycles of change, making small incremental steps to improve their lives. Also at this time she was working on a Robert Wood Johnson Foundation initiative that focused on interdisciplinary teamwork to improve care in pediatrics. Adding an interdisciplinary focus seemed to me to be key to unlocking the doors to improve quality in health care.

This was my turning point. I shared with her my interest in quality improvement. It was perfect timing as I was writing a John A. Hartford Foundation postdoctoral application. She creatively slipped into my post-doctoral plan quality improvement by adding attendance in the Metrohealth Medical Center Quality Scholars Program. Receiving the John A. Hartford Foundation award was my entrance into the world of quality! During this postdoctoral experience I attended weekly classes at MetroHealth on quality improvement and I also participated in the Cleveland Veterans Affairs National Quality Scholars program (VAQS), bimonthly educational sessions televised from Dartmouth University. My first project was on implementing alerts in the electronic medical record to improve diabetes care. Also during this postdoctoral experience I took Shirley's class, Continual Improvement in Healthcare: An Interdisciplinary Course. This course exposed me to a dynamic interdisciplinary faculty team (Linda Headrick and Duncan Neuhauser) and convinced me of the need to teach quality improvement concepts to frontline health care professionals.

After my postdoctoral experience, I was given the opportunity to use my quality improvement knowledge while leading the American Nurses Credentialing Center Magnet certification at University Hospitals Case Medical Center. During this project, I used my skills of teamwork, running effective meetings, and use of PDSA cycles. My emerging quality improvement philosophy guided me to take on this institutional project with confidence and skill. Shirley provided valuable guidance on the application of quality improvement in this project. It also was during this time that I experienced my first Institute for Healthcare Improvement National Forum, where I was inspired by Don Berwick.

In 2004, Shirley asked me to teach the quality improvement course along with an interdisciplinary team including Duncan Neuhauser, PhD; Nancy Tinsley, RN, MBA; and Mamta Singh, MD. Of course, Shirley provided valuable feedback for improving the course. We have continued the course, educating future leaders in health care to use the methods of quality improvement in their work. All students complete an interdisciplinary improvement project, and about 10% continue with improvement work by incorporating it into their final capstone project. Many of our students have obtained employment in quality – for example, working at the National Patient Safety Foundation, National Quality Forum, and the United States Public Health Service. One of our students has published her work, *State Tested Nursing Aides' Provision of End-of-Life Care in Nursing Homes: Implications for Quality Improvement*.[10]

It is incredible how the opportunities in quality improvement have been continuing through the work that Shirley ignited. Notably, I was asked to be the guest editor for the journal *Quality Management in Healthcare* with Dr. Mamta Singh. The issue highlighted the current state of quality improvement education. We also published a chapter in an international book, Quality Improvement and Chronic Health Conditions Implications for Research, in J. Ovretveit and P.J. Sousa's *Quality and Safety Improvement Research: Methods and Research Practice from the International Quality Improvement Research Network*.[11]

In 2008, I began my academic career at the Frances Payne Bolton School of Nursing. Shirley continued to mentor my quality journey. She negotiated with the dean for my appointment to lead the Quality and Safety Education for Nursing (QSEN) implementation project. We formed a team and developed an implementation plan to integrate the QSEN competencies into our baccalaureate, masters and doctoral programs at the school of nursing. The implementation model was published as a faculty resource on the QSEN website.[12] The QSEN journey continues at Frances Payne Bolton School of Nursing as Shirley and I will lead the National QSEN Institute marking the transition of the QSEN project from University of North Carolina to Case Western Reserve University.

Through Shirley's mentorship, in 2009 I was selected as the Cleveland VAQS Senior Fellow. In this role, I mentor nurses and physicians in improvement science in the now interprofessional VAQS program. To date, we have had five nurse pre- and postdoctoral fellows in the program. I also serve as a QSEN consultant, sharing my expertise in the implementation of the QSEN competencies into nursing curricula.

Other opportunities in which I have been involved include developing a quality improvement curriculum (web based) for the National State Boards of Nursing for their pilot of nurse residency programs, coauthoring a book with Shirley and colleagues on quality improvement for pre-licensure health care professionals, and coauthoring a chapter on interdisciplinary collaboration. Shirley's mentorship also has led to my involvement in three training grants that aim to increase interprofessional collaboration to improve quality and safety. Most notably, we worked together on a Robert Wood Johnson Foundation grant to improve the science of improvement by developing and testing an instrument to measure systems thinking, an important concept in quality improvement.

My incredible quality improvement journey continues and I am grateful for my mentor, Dr. Shirley Moore. She has provided opportunities to expand my quality improvement knowledge and skill and also connected me to people in quality improvement circles. Her greatest gift to me was her belief in me. This unattributed quote captures this element of mentorship: "A lot of people have gone further than they thought they could because someone else thought they could." Thank you, Shirley, for mentoring me like no other.

Reflections
....

Although the majority of this chapter is a personal reflection, by way of summary I will further reflect on what I am most proud of, what was most surprising, what I might do differently if I had the chance, and my dreams for the future.

What I am Most Proud Of

Over my career as a quality improvement educator, I am most proud of three things. First, I am incredibly pleased that the Interprofessional Healthcare Improvement course at CWRU has been ongoing for 18 years. Naturally, important changes have been made to the course – a next generation of better-trained faculty, the addition of content regarding safety in health care, and greater rigor in the teaching of statistical process control methods. The essentials of the course remain the same, however. It is still an interprofessional course taught by an interprofessional faculty; teams of learners continue to do hands-on improvement projects in local health care organizations; and an emphasis remains on engaging learners in cycles of action and reflection.

Second, I am proud of my leadership roles in QSEN and the VA Quality Scholars programs. Both programs are designing and evaluating new models of education for quality improvement in health care. Both have as their aim the development of a cadre of future health care professionals who will give care and also lead the improvement of care. I am proud of having provided leadership for these national quality improvement education initiatives that have influenced the lives of so many students and health care professionals who themselves have gone on to be leaders in the continual improvement of health care.

Third, I am very proud of having figured out a way to blend my interest and passion in quality improvement with my program of research in primary and secondary prevention of cardiovascular disease. Looking back now, it seems so clear. Health behaviors of individuals are a set of systems in their lives, and since all systems can be changed, one way to change health behavior systems is the use of process improvement techniques. Designing and testing a set of personal process improvement techniques for health behavior change has been a fruitful route for my research. When I started this journey in health care improvement, my fear was that it would interfere with my research program. It has turned out to the contrary; it has become a very successful element of my research.

What Was Most Surprising

The most surprising thing about my work in quality improvement education has been the extent to which I have applied the concepts of continuous quality improvement to other areas of my professional and personal life. In addition to my program of research, viewing the world from a more systems perspective has assisted me to understand the complexities of the academic and health care institutions in which I work. I appreciate the interdependencies inherent in my daily work and I have learned to acknowledge those interdependencies as I seek to promote change. In fact, I have found that many of the seemingly big changes I want to effect are best approached through a trial-and-error approach by applying a series of small experiments. I have found that people will try almost anything if it is viewed as a "pilot." I approach change in a hopeful, almost playful manner.

As I reflect on the nearly 20 years of my experience in quality improvement education, there have been some important changes in the US health care system that I believe have influenced the field of quality improvement education. One important change in the health care system is the shift to electronic health records and thus the availability of electronic databases containing information about processes, outcomes, and costs of care. The ability to examine the quality and costs of care of a population of patients at local, regional, and national levels provides the opportunity for better and faster understanding of how well we are improving the quality of care we give and assess any cost savings. Quality improvement educators now include the use of information systems as a major competency in quality improvement education. Another major shift over the past 20 years has been the emphasis on evidence-based practice. I am conflicted about whether or not this emphasis on evidence-based practice has helped or hurt the quality improvement movement, however. Although the use of evidence-based practice guidelines can certainly provide more standardized care and remove unwanted variation in care (central components of quality improvement), I note that practitioners often concentrate on their individual efforts to follow guidelines for treatment at the patient level, to the exclusion of addressing the underlying system issues in their care delivery systems that frequently play a crucial role in the delivery of high quality and safe care. I believe health professions educators have a considerable challenge to shift providers' traditional focus on the care of individual patients to taking responsibility for improving the systems of care in which they work.

What Would I Do Differently?

My reflection would not be complete without sharing what I would do differently if I had the chance. First, I would not have led such a "double life." For the first 8–10 years of my academic life I viewed quality improvement education as being "on the side." I had my mainstream focus on research and teaching in nursing, and considered my quality improvement education projects as being something separate or extra in which I was indulging because I liked the people I was working with and I enjoyed what I was doing. Even the quality improvement course that I was teaching was done as an unpaid overload in my teaching assignment. I was fearful that my work in the quality improvement education projects would be viewed as spending time on fringe projects, rather than concentrating on developing my program of research. After I received tenure and promotion to full professor, I became more relaxed about my quality improvement work. It is true also that the field of quality improvement in health care has advanced and become more mainstream in academia. Looking back, I think that the Institute of Medicine report *To Err is Human*[13] was the beginning of my "coming out." I hope that I have set in motion a new academic environment that embraces scholarship in quality and safety in health care.

My Dream for the Future

I need to confess that I have always thought of myself as a *creator of* history, not as a person who would be *reporting and reflecting on* history – in this case, the history of health professions education in quality improvement. So when asked to write this reflection on my experience as a leader in the field, I found it quite difficult. It is not hard for me, however, to share my images of the future of interprofessional education in quality and safety. The value of interprofessional education in health care has now been well documented. I plan to continue to champion interprofessional versus discipline-specific approaches to quality and safety education in the health professions. We still have a long way to go in terms of understanding how power differentials and the different mental models affect the delivery of high-quality health care.

A second goal I have is to help develop the next generation of researchers and scholars in the field of quality and safety. There have been few new theoretical approaches to quality improvement over the last 30 years. New theoretical approaches to quality and safety are needed. As a scholar, I worry that we have not challenged the existing paradigm of Deming, Batalden, Stolz, and others. I would like to see some head-to-head rigorous evaluations of different theoretical approaches to improving quality in health care.

In summary, I was asked in this chapter to describe my view of the changes in nursing education in quality and safety over the past 20 years. That has been difficult for me to do because I have viewed quality improvement education as an interdisciplinary process from the very beginning. I never set out to answer the question, "what will we teach nurses about quality improvement in health care?" My desire is for nurses to be informed and committed partners in health care quality improvement. My belief is that nurses can best achieve this through interdisciplinary education and I plan to continue my work to support this approach. Hmm, I wonder what small test of change I can do to test this belief in the next couple of weeks?

A Funny Thing Happened on the Way to the Forum (National Forum, Institute for Healthcare Improvement)

Mamta K. Singh, MD, MS
Associate Professor of Medicine, Case Western Reserve University School of Medicine
Physician Director, Center of Excellence in Primary Care Education

Louis Stokes Cleveland Veterans Affairs Medical Center Quality improvement education was the furthest from my mind when I started my residency in the mid-1990s. As with any first-year resident, the path to residency and then fellowship was set with the ultimate goal of being part of an academic practice. As dramatic as it sounds, one phone call changed all that. In the spring of my internship, I received a call from Dr. Linda Headrick, an esteemed faculty member of our General Medicine Division, asking that she would like to meet with me regarding career development opportunities. As a post-graduate year one resident, who could barely see past the call schedule, long-term career discussions seemed so abstract. The brief conversation did leave me intrigued – a new program in the General Medicine Division at MetroHealth Medical Center at Case Western Reserve University for future academic internists. It entailed completing a master's in health services research during one's internal medicine residency with a focus on longitudinal clinic experiences. It all sounded very attractive but so far off the beaten path. I signed up.

Fortunately for me, one of the first courses I took as part of my master's in health services research was Interdisciplinary Continuous Quality Improvement taught by Drs. Shirley Moore, Linda Headrick, Farrokh Alemi, and Duncan Neuhauser. As the semester progressed, I began to see clinical care in a different light and realized quickly that the traditional tools that I was given till this point were only partially preparing me to take care of my patients. If I wanted to take care of my patients the way I wanted to, something else was needed. The Quality Care Improvement class with these visionary educators was doing just that. Metaphorically, they were handing out new lenses and tools; no one graduated from the class ever seeing the health care world the same. Although this did result in a bit more angst at the daunting task of fixing systems and educating future health care professionals, it was coupled with an equal sense of empowerment that you could change things. Equipped with this drive, I began my journey in quality improvement education.

As I completed my residency and chief residency, I found myself using the model for improvement and rapid cycles of change for curriculum development and improvement. As a chief resident, I used small cycles of change to improve the daily Morning Report for our house staff and went on to publish the results of this improvement project. I attended and presented the Morning Report project at a workshop with Dr. Headrick at the National Institute for Health Care Improvement Forum in 1999. Immediately, I was struck by the energy and inspiration at the conference and it left a lasting mark. It was great to see thousands of people interested in making improvement in patient care systems so to provide better care. Hearing experts in the field such as Drs. Paul Batalden and Donald Berwick left no doubt in my mind that I had found my academic niche.

Given my interest in quality improvement, I was nominated and accepted into the Quality Faculty Scholars Program at MetroHealth for 2000–2001 (directed by Dr. Headrick). This was a hospital-wide faculty development program that allowed me to gain formal skills in quality improvement. My project focused on improving the screening and treatment of patients with osteoporosis. As the team leader of this initiative, I played an integral role in bringing different departments together to improve bone density results reporting by radiology and subsequently created a "Smart Set" template order for osteoporosis in the electronic medical record system.

My clinical interests in women's health coupled with my successes in using the quality improvement infrastructure led to my chair asking me to start a women's health clinic. Building on my experience in bringing together diverse groups, I was able to get departmental faculty from Obstetrics/Gynecology and Internal Medicine together to develop a women's health curriculum. (At that time, this was what I thought it was to be interprofessional!) We established a mandatory ambulatory clinic for internal medicine residents, which focused on preventive health education while providing key services to female patients. Not only was this clinic very popular with residents as measured by surveys, but we also demonstrated improved clinical outcomes in cervical cancer screening.[14] This was in keeping with the quality improvement mantra; it is not enough to just provide care, one should always be thinking of how to improve it.[15] The clinic model was presented at local and national meetings and I received the Scholarship in Teaching Award for this work by Case Western Reserve University (CWRU).

In 2004, I expanded my interests in medical education into the undergraduate medical curriculum as part of CWRU's Primary Care Track and then moved on to direct pre-clerkship patient-based programs for all CWRU medical students. Not only did this leadership role result in important avenues of collaboration and learning at the medical school, but also it provided me with a unique opportunity to marry my expertise in quality with medical education in community practices. The result was two US Department of Health and Human Services Health Resources and Services Administration grants, which continue to provide an important source of intellectual stimulus as well as hard-to-come-by extramural support for education. Quality improvement web modules developed as part of this effort have also been recognized with a CWRU Scholarship in Teaching award.

My engagement at the medical school has also provided a wealth of opportunity to design, support, and implement a comprehensive series of quality and patient safety educational initiatives that span the entire curriculum. This includes a longitudinal quality improvement (QI) curriculum in years one and two and interprofessional patient safety sessions in the year three curriculum. I have also participated in the Harvard Macy Program for Educators in the Health Professions,[16] with a project aimed at expanding a more comprehensive QI curriculum to the third year. (The Harvard Macy Program is described further in Chapter 2 of this volume, "From Freedom to Learn to Freedom to Innovate: The Harvard Macy Institute Story," by Elizabeth G. Armstrong with Sylvia Barsion.) At the same time I was invited to participate in a working group for the school's Prentiss Grant on the development of a patient safety and quality curriculum, participating in several retreats and helping to write an entirely new series of questions for the National Board of Medical Examiners United States Medical Licensing Examination Step 1 and Step 2 exams.[17]

As I worked at designing and studying ways to introduce health care quality into medical education, I became increasingly aware of the lack of rigor in QI learning evaluation schemes and the need to align these with learning goals. My interest in this area, along with a desire to take my academic career to the next level with intensive focus and mentorship, led me to make a career shift and enroll as a fellow in the Veterans Affairs Quality Scholars Fellowship Program.[18] As I furthered my QI expertise through the Scholars program, the interdisciplinary nature of QI has provided the opportunity to build on my prior interprofessional experience and work closely with colleagues at the School of Nursing. Here I returned to work with nationally recognized quality improvement educators such as Dr. Shirley Moore. This collaborative work resulted in being a coinvestigator with principal investigators Drs. Mary Dolansky and Shirley Moore on the Robert Wood Johnson Foundation-funded study to develop and validate an instrument to measure systems thinking. As a result of this interdisciplinary collaboration, the Institute for Health Care Improvement/Macy Foundation chose CWRU as one of six demonstration sites to pilot undergraduate QI interdisciplinary learning where I was coprincipal investigator along with my colleague in nursing, Dr. Deborah Lindell. The collaboration efforts have also afforded me the opportunity to guest edit the *Quality Management in Health Care* journal (July, 2009) with Dr. Mary Dolansky, dedicated to quality improvement in education; to organize and moderate the Quality Improvement Summit held at CWRU in October 2009; and to participate in the US Department of Veteran Affairs' national initiative on Patient-Centered Medical Home training and evaluation. Now I am the physician director of the Cleveland Veterans Affairs Medical Center's Center of Excellence in Primary Care Education, a 5-year, 5-million-dollar funded project.[19] I find this program has been particularly satisfying for me. It has provided an excellent platform to align my interests in quality improvement education, general internal medicine, and health services research while allowing me to explore and develop robust measurement and assessment systems.

Many colleagues and faculty questioned whether I would be able to make a career out of quality improvement. Perhaps it is a fad and as with all fads, what are you going to do when it no longer is considered glamorous? Over the last 12 years I have been fortunate to be able to build on my training in general internal medicine and health services research to develop a career focus that brings together medical education, health care quality, and interprofessional collaboration. These are themes that are not only important for the ongoing development of curriculum but also critical to the evolution of our national health care system. The opportunities for innovation and scholarship are expanding dramatically and drawing increasing recognition from funding agencies at all levels. There is much more work to do – I feel I have positioned myself well to be an active participant in this exciting environment both locally and nationally. Funny, to think it all began with a phone call.

References

1. Headrick LA, Knapp M, Neuhauser D, *et al.* Working from upstream to improve health care: the IHI Interdisciplinary Professional Education Collaborative. *Jt Comm J Qual Improv.* 1996; **22**(3): 149–64.
2. Senge P. *The Fifth Discipline: The Art and Practice of the Learning Organization.* New York, NY: Doubleday/Currency; 1990.
3. Cronenwett L, Sherwood G, Gelmon SB. Improving quality and safety education: the QSEN Learning Collaborative. *Nurs Outlook.* 2009; **57**(6): 304–12.
4. Cronenwett L, Sherwood G, Pohl J, *et al.* Quality and safety education for advanced nursing practice. *Nurs Outlook.* 2009; **57**(6): 338–48.
5. Sherwood G. Integrating quality and safety science in nursing education and practice. *J Res Nurs.* 2011; **16**(3): 226–40.
6. Sherwood G, Barnsteiner J, editors. *Quality and Safety in Nursing: A Competency Approach to Improving Outcomes.* Hoboken, NJ: Wiley-Blackwell; 2012.
7. Splaine ME, Ogrinc G, Gilman SC, *et al.* The Department of Veterans Affairs National

Quality Scholars Fellowship Program: experience from 10 years of training quality scholars. *Acad Med.* 2009; **84**(12): 1741–8.

8. www.a4hi.org
9. Alemi F, Neuhauser D. *A Thinking Person's Step by Step Guide to Weight Loss and Exercise Program.* Victoria, BC: Trafford Publishing; 2005.
10. Nochomovitz E, Prince-Paul MJ, Dolansky MA, *et al.* State tested nursing aides' provision of end-of-life care in nursing homes: implications for quality improvement. *J Hosp Palliat Nurs.* 2010; **12**(4): 255–62.
11. Neuhauser D, Dolansky MA, Singh M. Quality improvement and chronic health conditions implications for research. In: Øvretveit J, Sousa PJ, editors. *Quality and Safety Improvement Research: Methods and Research Practice from the International Quality Improvement Research Network.* Lisbon, Portugal: Alfanumérico; 2008. pp. 57–64.
12. *Quality and Safety Education for Nurses. Module 9: Managing Curricular Change for QSEN Integration. Faculty Resources.* Available at: http://qsen.org/faculty-resources/learning-modules/ (accessed February 28, 2013).
13. Institute of Medicine. *To Err is Human: Building a Better Health System.* Washington, DC: National Academies Press; 2000.
14. Singh MK, Einstadter D, Lawrence R. A structured women's preventive health clinic for residents: a quality improvement project designed to meet training needs and improve cervical cancer screening rates. *Qual Saf Health Care.* 2010; **19**(5): e45.
15. Batalden P, Davidoff F. Teaching quality improvement: the devil is in the details. *JAMA.* 2007; **298**(9): 1059–61.
16. *Program for Educators in the Health Professions.* Boston, MA: Harvard Macy Institute; 2012. Available at: www.harvardmacy.org/programs/Programs-Educators.aspx (accessed February 28, 2013).
17. *USMLE: For Students and Graduates of Medical Schools in the United States and Canada Accredited by the LCME or AOA.* Philadelphia, PA: National Board of Medical Examiners; 2011. Available at: www.nbme.org/students/usmle.html (accessed October 5, 2012).
18. *VA Quality Scholars Fellowship Program.* Washington, DC: United States Department of Veterans Affairs; 2012. Available at: www.va.gov/oaa/specialfellows/programs/SF_NQSF_default.asp (accessed October 5, 2012).
19. *VA Centers of Excellence in Primary Care Education.* Washington, DC: United States Department of Veterans Affairs; 2011. Available at: www.va.gov/oaa/rfp_Coe.asp (accessed October 5, 2012).

11

Reforming Medical Education
Confessions of a Battered Humanist

DeWitt C. Baldwin Jr.

WHEN IT COMES TO REFORMING MEDICAL EDUCATION, ONE PROBABLY does well to remember the French admonition *plus ça change, plus c'est la même chose* – the more things change, the more they are the same! As sociologist Sam Bloom has insightfully pointed out, despite the frequent calls for reform in medical education, most of the intended changes in the curriculum over the past century have ended up being essentially "change without reform," since the underlying conceptual models, ideologies, values, and culture of undergraduate medical education have not been fundamentally altered.[1] This observation was recently echoed by medical historian Ken Ludmerer,[2] who stated that despite the many expert panel reports over the years, little real change has occurred in the basic conceptual model and practice of graduate medical education. These observations would seem to suggest that significant reforms in medical education still await transformative and paradigmatic shifts in conceptual models of education and organizational culture.[3]

Conception and Birth of an Educational Innovation

In 1970, after 20 years on the faculties of four traditional and two new medical schools, I decided to leave medicine. For years, my aim had been to try to "humanize" medical education and patient care, believing that "As teacher is to student, doctor will be to patient." In the early 1950s, I had taught medical and other health professional students at an interprofessional Child Health Clinic at the University of Washington. And I felt some appreciation for my efforts when students told me, "Other doctors teach us what to *do to* patients. You teach us how to *be with* patients." What I soon discovered, of course, was that medical education was remarkably resistant to change, with universal acceptance of the traditional lockstep march through 2 years of basic sciences followed by 2 years of clinical sciences.[4] Moreover, it seemed difficult to question a system that had been in place for many years and seemed to be doing a pretty good job. Yet what was clear was that medical education was standing still, while health care and the practice of medicine were changing radically, with a shift in the focus of care from acute to chronic illness, and increasing recognition that a range of factors impact health, including poverty, social class, gender, and race.

From 1950 to 1980, some 40 new medical schools were started in the United States, many espousing a community-based focus.[5] During this same period, at least two major educational curriculum designs were introduced into the basic sciences: the *organ-system* approach at Case-Western Reserve and the *problem-based* curriculum at McMaster in Canada. Despite these examples of educational innovation, however, one of my greatest frustrations was the difficulty I and others were experiencing in trying to introduce into the curriculum the newly relevant knowledge and skills from the social and behavioral sciences, ethics, economics, and the humanities.[6] As Bloom and others have pointed out, the problem here was to think that the curriculum was the fulcrum for change, when the fault lay with underlying ideology and culture.[1]

Especially difficult to accept was that after innovative and idealistic beginnings, even the "new" schools with which I was associated soon looked exactly like the traditional ones. Part of this was because the available pool of medical faculty had themselves all been educated in the traditional system. Another was the resistance of the Liaison Committee on Medical Education (LCME) at that time to any substantial change in the system.

Because of my interest in child development, I decided to go back to teaching early childhood education, a time in life when learning is natural, engaged in for its own sake, and embraced with energy and enthusiasm. At the last second, however, in 1971, I was asked to help start my third new medical school, this time at the University of Nevada, Reno – one so new (I was on the planning group), so small (nine full-time faculty), and so impoverished, both financially (our first check from the state was for $14 000!) and scientifically (hand-me-down and borrowed faculty, courses, equipment, space, and resources), that there didn't seem to be much for people to fight over or room for any pretensions. Among other things, the small size meant that traditional "departments" of this or that science were out of the question. The new school was organized into three small divisions – Basic Sciences, Behavioral Sciences, and Clinical Sciences, and took over an old science building located next to the Nursing School.

The Anatomy of an Innovation

The attraction of the new medical school for me was the possibility of creating rather than trying to change an existing system. The Legislative Act creating the 2-year medical school at the University of Nevada, Reno, had authorized an "interdisciplinary" Health Sciences Program that included preprofessional undergraduate education. I immediately saw the opportunity to introduce and integrate my long-term educational passions, social and behavioral sciences, early patient and community contact, and interprofessional education and teamwork early into the mainstream of medical education. I leapt at the opportunity to lead this effort. I quickly figured that if we could extend some of my ideas (especially the social and behavioral sciences) into preprofessional education, students' outlook on medicine and the other professions might be quite different. So while I originally came to head the Division of Behavioral Sciences in the medical school, I also wound up leading the new Interdisciplinary Health Sciences Program on the undergraduate university campus. To assist this effort, I secured a major grant from the Robert Wood Johnson Foundation (RWJF) to assemble a unique interprofessional faculty who could help me plan, design, implement, and teach a complete interprofessional health sciences curriculum that would be required of all preprofessional students planning to enter the health field at the University, which would extend through professional education.

In the early 1970s, the term "interdisciplinary" was used throughout higher education. In 1975, Rosemary Kane's seminal monograph on "Interprofessional Teamwork" proposed that these two terms be used in place of "interdisciplinary" and "team."[7] The term interprofessional is now accepted internationally and will be used throughout the rest of this chapter.

The following excerpt is the opening paragraph of the grant proposal to the Robert Wood Johnson Foundation, 1972.

Although increasing emphasis is placed on the role of the interdisciplinary team in health care delivery, students enrolled in medicine, nursing, and the other health professions and occupations traditionally have little contact with one another in the process of their education and still less planned collaborative learning experience designed to promote such relationships. Upon graduation, however, they are expected to work effectively with one another in the community.

Building the Preprofessional, Interprofessional Education Prototype

Nevada proved to be uniquely positioned for imaginative educational innovations. A conservative state, paradoxically, it turned out to be a place where "the utterly rational might take forever, but the utterly impossible could happen tomorrow." By its own Statement of Philosophy, the fledgling medical school came onto the campus committed, not only to the entire "continuum "of medical education including preprofessional education, but to the statement, "It is essential to plan for interdisciplinary experiences in health team relationships."

The new preprofessional interprofessional education (IPE) core curriculum had a *horizontal*, lower division component comprised of all the university and preprofessional biomedical requirements. To conserve resources and facilitate interprofessional learning, we asked the university science departments to revise their basic science service courses to better interest and serve the special needs of the health sciences students, rather than just their own majors, with redesigned courses, such as Life Sciences Chemistry and Biochemistry and Human Anatomy and Physiology. These rapidly gained high enrollments, which pleased the Science Departments. Since such courses served all the health sciences students, they were truly interprofessional. This also meant that all preprofessional students would have the advantage of later occupational mobility, since they shared the same science requirements.

> For a more detailed description of the content, structure, process, and development of the prototype interprofessional education curriculum described, please see an article (originally published in *Medical Education Since 1960: Marching to a Different Drummer*,[8] 1979) reprinted in 2007 as part of a supplement of the *Journal of Interprofessional Care*, **21**(Suppl. 1): 52–69.

Meanwhile, a special *vertical* core was created across all four preprofessional years aimed at providing a planned sequence of eight required and eight elective interprofessional, team-taught, and team learning experiences, involving both the classroom and the community. These covered all the common knowledge areas shared by the nine health sciences programs then on campus: medical terminology, bioethics, nutrition, pharmacology, communication skills, growth and development, death and dying, social and behavioral sciences, family and community health, wellness, human sexuality, health education, health care systems, health economics, and team delivery of care. These courses were designed to be taught in a unique, experiential way.

The interprofessional teamwork theme was integrated into everything we did in the IPE curriculum. From day one, we tried to orient our teaching inventively around this theme by setting up multiple, small group, problem-based learning exercises in the classroom, as well as team-based community projects. On the very first day of class, for example, entering health sciences students were seated around tables of eight, with no more than one representative from any future health profession. After introducing themselves they were facilitated in exploring their perceptions and expectations of their own vocational choices and those of others. (By the way, not the least of the institutional barriers to IPE at the university level was the difficulty finding level, open-space classrooms with movable tables and chairs, where such informal learning could take place.)

Educational methods included dyadic, triadic, and small group exercises and activities, simulations, role-plays, team games, group projects and field assignments aimed at enhancing knowledge of and attitudes toward members of the other health professions. Evaluation was likewise unique, much of it linked to group projects, employing self and peer evaluations. We even instituted detailed student evaluations of the faculty and teaching methods, a novelty at that time (and information that we listened to!). The objective was to fully explore and develop knowledge about the health professions in the classroom and in the community, along with concepts of health and wellness, self-awareness, and values clarification, as well as goal-setting, problem solving, decision making, and leadership – all basic skills for team building.

In the second or sophomore year, the focus was on practical skills development. Working again in dyads, triads, and simulated interprofessional teams, students learned psychosocial communication and medical interviewing skills, as well as physical, social, nutritional, and developmental assessment, including emergency medical assessment and intervention (students were enabled to become emergency medical technicians), involving community agencies and personnel.

The third-year courses focused on in-depth studies of the health care system, health policy and economics, and health care delivery, including cost, quality, and accessibility, as well as human values, biomedical ethics, and professional behavior. Wherever possible, students were expected to conduct projects or investigate these issues in classroom or community settings in small groups or on simulated teams. It is of some note that the junior level course in bioethics in 1972 may have been among the first offered at any institution of higher learning in the United States.

As seniors expecting to graduate with baccalaureate degrees in their chosen professions, students were introduced to topics like gerontology, human sexuality, and death and dying. They were also expected to participate on interprofessional student clinical teams, representing their own professions, together with medical students, providing health maintenance and care for selected families under the supervision of our faculty interprofessional teams at the primary care and geriatric clinics sponsored by the program.

Because the core courses were required, the number of students enrolled in the Health Sciences Program grew rapidly until nearly one-sixth of all students attending the university (over 1000 were enrolled by 1975) created a demanding logistic scheduling problem for the faculty. Some of this was alleviated by using advanced students as teaching assistants, as well as health professionals from the community. One of our early lessons was that the entire team did not have to all be at the front of the classroom or leading an exercise at the same time and that much of the teamwork occurred during preparation.

> The good thing about the Health Sciences Program is that it happens at a time when the students are susceptible to change – when they are first beginning to form their attitudes. It's neat because they don't have all these preconceived ideas about what a nurse is or does, or a social worker is or does.
>
> *—Marcus Erling, premedical student,*
> *University of Nevada, Reno (recorded on film, 1976)*

> It was an exciting time – vibrant, collegial, resonant, good teaching, non-competitive, we saw other professions, and learned ethics. Entry to med school was seamless. I entered primary care. I didn't realize till later how good the program was.
>
> *—Dr. Marcus Erling, Las Vegas, Nevada*
> *(personal communication, February 15, 2012)*

A Unique Intercultural, Interprofessional Service-Learning Experience

Nevada had another interesting feature. A frontier state, the nation's seventh largest, it contained 23 Native American Reservations. Because of their number and wide distribution, as well as limited Indian Health Service resources and personnel, there were enormous unmet health needs on the reservations. What an opportunity for unique field placement experiences for health sciences students to provide health services while learning to work together as teams, as well as for developing communication and intercultural skills. A grant from the federal government, designed specifically to train student interprofessional teams in primary care, built upon the IPE curriculum above by providing opportunities for advanced team training for the Health Sciences undergraduates during summer and spring vacations.

Supervised by our IPE faculty teams, interested advanced health professions students and first- and second-year medical students (we were still a 2-year school) were assigned to primary care teams which visited tribal reservations in the state to conduct developmental and health assessments, as well as hypertension and diabetes screenings and case findings. After a week of intensive training covering medical, team building, and intercultural issues, the teams went "circuit-riding" to their assigned reservations. Since one of the major issues was acceptance of the "anglo" teams on the reservations, we also recruited Native American students from the university with an interest in the health field to participate on the student teams, "shadowing" a different health professional student each day, and being encouraged to try interventions, such as history taking, nutritional assessment, and conducting vision and hearing tests. One often saw the health professions students teaching the Native American students how to take blood pressures and conducting eye and hearing tests. Their presence really made the visits a success from every standpoint. Several of the medical students who participated in this program later served in the Indian Health Service.[9]

My Other Job: Nevada's New Medical School

Meanwhile, starting out at the medical school, I was a one-person Division of Behavioral Sciences, whereas in the previous year at Connecticut I had had an outstanding group of ten double-degree, social and behavioral sciences faculty. With help from my social worker wife and a psychologist on sabbatical, I asked for and got the first day of the curriculum with the medical students. I designed it to be an experiential, humanizing experience where students and faculty could share their hopes, desires, expectations, and concerns about the road ahead (besides being a new school, it was only approved for the first 2 years). Were they good enough to succeed? Were we? The small size of the class, 32, really helped. Between our enthusiasm and theirs, and a mutual willingness to take things as they came, we evolved quickly into a family. We all wanted to make it work.

I campaigned for early clinical and community contact, and the students were assigned to visit local physicians' offices from the start. I also got a regular chunk of time each week for teaching my other love, the social and behavioral sciences. Since we did not have the faculty resources I'd had elsewhere, I decided to teach in small groups of 12 and to make our sessions essentially problem-based and experiential. I offered my small group a chance to experience patients early and close up, by offering them training and arranging for them to take night call on a community crisis hot line. Between that and their visits to physicians' offices, we had lots to talk about at our weekly group sessions. Substantive questions were referred back to the group and reprints made available. Also, personal and professional friends (it was amazing how many people found Reno interesting!), such as Dame Cicely Saunders (Hospice), Elizabeth Kubler Ross (Death and Dying), Frederic Leboyer (Birth without Violence), Sir John Fry, the Queen's physician (British National Health Service), Sol Levine (Medical Sociology), Virginia Satir (Family Therapy), Richard Bandler and John Grinder (Neurolinguistic Programming), and Ivan Illich ("Medical Nemesis"), all met with students.

We expanded the early clinical contact idea further by starting to teach clinical skills in the fall semester of the first year with instruction and practice in interviewing and communication skills, moving into physical examination skills after Christmas. Nothing did more to cement the idea that we were a "family" than when students needed to learn to do pelvic examinations, and my wife and several of our IPE nurse faculty volunteered. I've never seen such respectful and appreciative students in my life! When these first-year students went on their doctors' office visits in the spring, local physicians remarked that they seemed more like residents than students. As noted earlier, when clinical interprofessional team experiences were offered to our preprofessional students, the medical students were likewise invited.

The basic sciences faculty began using an organ system approach, pairing our limited faculty with physicians in the community. By the end of their second year, our students all did well on the National Board exams, and my small group method in the behavioral sciences resulted in scores much higher than the national average (even though the students had earlier complained to the dean that I had never "taught" them anything!). More importantly, when we transferred our students into the third year at other medical schools across the country, a number later graduated at the top of their new classes. At least three students from these early years went on to become deans of medical schools and two are currently chancellors of the health science universities in their states.

I had a superb experience in that first class at the medical school. In that first semester, I took crisis call (after training), a 24-hour marathon T-group with you, learned medical interviewing, attended workshops with some of the visiting faculty like family therapist, Virginia Satir, participated in the weekly support groups at your house with grad students from other fields, including my future wife, who was a graduate nursing student, and saw patients in my preceptor's office. The small numbers of students, early clinical contact, faculty who really cared about us and helped us explore medicine with excitement were key. You and the faculty helped me "grow up." The behavioral and social side of medicine made me a better student, physician and person. I was very well prepared for my transfer to Emory in the 3rd year, as well as for residency and practice. I can't thank you enough.

—Dr. James Moren, member of first medical school class at Nevada; currently a family practitioner working with an interprofessional health care team at the local Veterans Administration clinic in Bellingham, Washington (personal communication, January 9, 2012)

Educational Philosophy of the Interprofessional Education Curriculum

Our educational philosophy was closely patterned on what today is sometimes described as andragogy, or adult learning theory: learner-focused, experiential, small group, and problem-based. I had learned this educational approach from my parents, who were pioneers in adult education during the 1930s. When they returned from 10 years as educational missionaries in Burma in 1933 with the belief that "we have as much to learn as we have to teach," they were promptly fired by their Mission Board. In response, they proceeded to interview college and graduate students across the United States, finding them to be extraordinarily isolationist and provincial (and not likely to support foreign missions!).

The Board promptly rehired them, but instead of "preaching" (the Board's expectation) about what my parents were calling "world-mindedness," they designed and implemented a program for experientially teaching it. They did this by conducting experiential, residential, international, interracial, intercultural, interfaith, service-learning workshops in the summers, starting in 1936, that featured many of the principles and methods we later employed with our Nevada students.

> "Conceptually, my parents were real pioneers in education. They believed in "experiential learning" – that learning is best keyed to the immediate needs of the learner and is grounded in real-life situations and tasks. In addition, they believed in the principle of "alternation" in learning – periods of intense learning experience followed by times for reflection and integration.[10] They also believed in learning through service, and my father is listed, along with John Dewey and Paulo Freire, as one of the pioneers of "service-learning."[11] Finally, they were pioneers in small group learning and in group dynamics, utilizing "diversity" of experience and viewpoint within the group as ways to challenge and transform fixed ideas and assumptions. They presciently even called their summer, live-in, service-learning working experience "a laboratory experience in human relations" (in the 1930s!)."
>
> —*DeWitt C. Baldwin, Jr.*
> *October, 2007[12]*

With this background (I participated in these experiences during my high school and college summers), it is no wonder that I became interested in education, experiential learning, small-group dynamics, and adult learning theory.

Having committed ourselves to the value and effectiveness of experiential learning, diversity, small-group dynamics, self-discovery, and service-learning, we tried to treat our students as adult learners and "colleagues in learning." We aspired to be "guides on the side, rather than sages on the stage." It may sound strange, but the whole program was so radical and exciting that we on the faculty often felt as if we were learning as much as the students.

It should be apparent by now that the interprofessional Health Sciences Program at Nevada espoused a totally different educational philosophy than was usually found at other universities and health professions schools at the time. Certainly it was vastly different from the rest of the Nevada campus. In fact, such adult learning educational ideas are still clearly contrary to the way most universities teach and it's not surprising that they are frequently viewed as subversive. No wonder we were regarded as rebels. We came in for considerable criticism as being too liberal and giving too much responsibility to the students. At times, this translated into experiencing a lot of difficulty getting our courses approved. A lot of this probably was envy of our resources and our evident success with the students, who seemed to enjoy our educational philosophy and methods. We often defensively referred to our program as "our island of sanity," realizing, however, that at times, it served to set us apart from the rest of the campus.

Not only did we believe in and practice the empowerment of students, we also practiced empowerment for our faculty. Members were encouraged and enabled to take time off for self and professional development. Time was arranged for securing advanced degrees and no less than eight full-time IPE faculty members were able to get advanced degrees while serving in the program. Four received their professional doctorates, three of them using the IPE program for their dissertation topics. To keep ourselves on target, we held faculty development sessions each Friday, featuring a sit-down lunch, as well as a staff meeting, often with an outside consultant or a planned educational exercise in team-building. Unique features of our meetings were the presence of a "process observer/

It was a heady time – a real "Camelot" experience for many of us. I have pictures in my mind as if it were yesterday – sitting in your office writing a grant or planning the next step and feeling valued and important as a colleague with complete respect for my (our) ideas and participation. You were a guide on the side, but also a sage in what we were trying to do. You had a real "greatness" of Being.

—*Linda Peterson, PhD, Emeritus Professor, University of Nevada School of Medicine, and Pediatric nurse practitioner and psychologist on the original Health Science Program / interprofessional education faculty team (personal communication, January 16, 2012)* timekeeper," who was tasked with keeping us focused and on time, a rotating "Devil's Advocate," who was charged with questioning the assumptions and decisions of the group, and the regular use of the NASA Action Item Log (originally used by the Space Program to keep track of action items by assigning dates and persons responsible).

Evaluation and Research

We included money and positions in the RWJF grant, described earlier, for a research and evaluation team. They supplied regular formative and summative evaluation of the program, students, and faculty. There is insufficient space for more than a mention, but our sophisticated research program is summarized in an article describing this innovation.[8,13] In particular, however, I want to mention the very sophisticated, forward-looking research on Interaction Analysis[14,15] conducted by Dr. Barbara Thornton, who received her PhD for studying the patterns of communication and interaction on our own student and faculty teams.

Finally, I want to add what may be among the more significant outcomes in terms of current workforce needs. Since we had two streams of entering medical students, those who had participated in our undergraduate interprofessional program (IPE), and those from traditional pre-med programs at our own and other universities, we could compare the effect of an early IPE experience with regard to their eventual specialty choices. Data from Nevada's medical graduates from 1977 to 1980 disclosed that of the 61 medical students who had participated as preprofessionals or professionals in our IPE program during those years, 80% (n = 49) later selected a primary care specialty, while only 44% (n = 51) of the 115 students from the traditional pre-medical sciences backgrounds made such a selection (Baldwin, unpublished data).

The Price One Can Pay for Innovation

We eventually paid a price for this freedom, experimentation, and separateness. By 1980, when federal grant funding began drying up, making our case for permanent state support became increasingly difficult. Even though our courses had developed more than nine FTEs (full-time faculty equivalents), we were only credited with three FTEs by the university, mainly for our lower division courses, and totally insufficient to support our important upper-level, clinical interprofessional team curriculum. Furthermore, applications for tenure for our IPE faculty, while approved by the medical school (by now the IPE program had been attached to the Medical School as the Division of Health Sciences), were being denied by the University.

In addition to the changing fiscal situation, there were important administrative changes. The three original campus deans who had birthed the Health Sciences Program had all moved on or retired. There also had been three deans of the Medical School, four college presidents, and in 1983, I left to become President of Earlham College in Richmond, Indiana. Back in Nevada, a new College of Health and Human Services was formed, incorporating the old Health Sciences Program and its lower level courses.

By this time, the medical school had become a success. We had secured state approval and funding to expand to a fully accredited 4-year school in 1978, a fact that further alienated the rest of the university, which also needed additional resources. As part of the expansion of the medical school, our innovative idea of staying small and creating only a Division of Primary Care (comprising the clinical specialties of Family Medicine, Pediatrics and Internal Medicine) and a Division of Specialty Care (including the rest of the specialties), which seemed to make so much sense for a small school like ours, was denied by the LCME accreditation agency. Instead, Nevada was required to follow the traditional path of recruiting expensive clinical departments of "this and that" specialty at a time when financial resources were becoming a constraining factor throughout health care and medical education.

This did open up a fortuitous evolutionary move for the main body of our clinical interprofessional faculty team, however, which simply moved into the medical school as the new Family Medicine Department, continuing their existing clinical and educational activities, unfortunately, now mostly for medical students. Except for two members of the IPE faculty, who filled the available University positions and continued to teach a few of the core IPE Courses (my daughter took some of them in the mid-1990s), the rest of the faculty moved on to positions elsewhere, at least one to the new geriatric IP training programs being developed nationally at VA Hospitals.

Flash! Breaking News

It is indeed ironic that in 2010, the University of Nevada, Reno announced the establishment of an "innovative" new Division of Health Sciences, charged with implementing interprofessional educational experiences for medical, nursing, and other health sciences students! By the way, did I mention that patience and a sense of humor are also useful qualities for an innovator?

> I'm amazed to find that life has brought me back full circle to where I began forty years ago. Just last week, I was asked to teach in the "new" Health Sciences program now developing on the UNR [University of Nevada, Reno] campus.
>
> —*Linda Peterson, RN, PhD, Emeritus Professor, University of Nevada School of Medicine (personal communication, January 16, 2012)*

What Was Going on Elsewhere in Interprofessional Education?
• • • • • • • • • • • • • • •

In the late 1960s and early 1970s, there was a lot of interest in "interdisciplinary" collaboration and team health care in the United States. This was largely as a result of President Johnson's Great Society Program and the resultant Community Health Center movement, where interprofessional primary care teams were being touted as the best way to deliver much-needed health care to rural and urban underserved populations. The problematic experiences of these early teams led leaders such as Harold Wise, Director of the Dr. Martin Luther King Health Center in New York, to turn to Professor Richard Beckhard and his group from the Sloan School of Management at the Massachusetts Institute of Technology to better understand the dynamics of teams and teamwork. Their studies were published and are still a standard for the field.[16–18]

Along with the widespread student protests of this period nationally, an important, but little remembered, piece was the activism of the student health organizations which formed in the late 1960s (including later, the American Medical Student Association) in response to the dissatisfaction of medical, dental, nursing, and other health science students with the way they were being educated.[19] They managed to garner support for deploying interdisciplinary student health teams to work with rural and urban underserved populations. By 1975, it was estimated that some 5000 students had participated in such interdisciplinary, service-learning, experiences across the nation. (R. Merrill, personal communication, 1995.)

At Montefiore Hospital in New York, an early adopter, David Kindig,[20] and others formed the Institute for Health Team Development, an interprofessional consulting and practice group. Kindig shortly was asked to head up a new Federal Office of Interdisciplinary Programs at the Health Resources and Services Administration in Washington. There he secured funding to train health professions students in team care at a select group of universities, including the University of Nevada, Reno.

A High Point of Interprofessional Education Interest in the United States

In 1976, I was invited by Dorothy Rouse of the Office of Interdisciplinary Programs to set up a conference at Snowbird, Utah, designed to glean the early experiences and successes and problems in student health care team training at the funded university programs. I would have to say that the Snowbird conference probably represented the high point of IPE and student team training up until this time in the United States. Nearly every knowledgeable person in the field was assembled at this conference to learn from the experiences of the funded schools and to try to develop a state-of-the-art working theory of IPE team training. As cohost, Nevada published the summary report,[21] which was later reprinted by the University of Kentucky in 1982.

In an effort to continue this exchange of information and experience, another of the funded schools, the University of Washington, hosted a conference in 1979, where a full program of papers was presented. Eight of 19 presentations (four of eight of these on research) were from our program and the University of Nevada again published what became the Proceedings of this First Interdisciplinary Health Care Team Conference (IHCTC) in 1980. This began a tradition that continued until 2003, with annual conferences hosted largely by universities with an interest in IPE and interprofessional practice (IPP), and orchestrated by a volunteer "executive" committee. There was never a formal organization of any kind and the effort was supported on a volunteer basis. Sadly, I estimate that more than 500 worthwhile papers on IPE and IPP were published in these Proceedings over the years and are essentially lost to the indexed literature, as there was no interest on the part of the traditional professional journals in this topic at the time.

> Bud is one of the real pioneers of interprofessionalism in health care and inter-professional education in the USA, having started his active practice of both in the early 1950s at the University of Washington. By the time I met him, he had already created a complete, required, four-year, pre-professional, interdisciplinary health team training core curriculum at the University of Nevada, Reno (UNR) in the early 1970s. When fully developed, over a thousand undergraduate students in nine different health care disciplines were enrolled, a curricular feat that remains unduplicated in the United States to the present day.
>
> When Bud and I met, the annual IHCTC conferences that he and his colleagues had initiated were the only forums for interprofessional discussions among educators, clinicians, and researchers across the health disciplines in the US. He was friendly and enthusiastic, supporting others to step into leadership roles to keep IHCTC going – ultimately for 24 years. Four of us – all nurses on the faculty of the University of Rochester School of Nursing – attended the 3rd IHCT conference. He was personally encouraging of our theoretically driven collaborative research projects on the outcomes of interdisciplinary health care team interventions, which he recognized were needed in this new field. From that time on, it has been my privilege to be a mentee, colleague, coauthor, and close friend of Bud's, joining legions of others whom he has influenced professionally and personally.
>
> —*Madeline Schmitt RN, PhD, FAAN Professor Emerita,*
> *University of Rochester School of Nursing, Rochester, New York*
> *(personal communication, January 18, 2012)*

This intense flame of interest in IPE began to fade starting in 1980, when fiscal constraints led to the end of federal funding for these programs. I sometimes think that the IPE movement in the United States might have died then except for the fact that the Veterans Administration suddenly became aware of the growing problem of aging veterans and their increasing needs for comprehensive health services involving multiple health professions, and undertook a long-term program of interprofessional geriatric team training. In addition, some federal funding continued for interprofessional training in federal programs for area health education centers and in rural health.

International Interest in Interprofessional Education

I had support from the Milbank Fund in 1968 to visit a number of European countries to learn about interprofessional education, at that time involving medicine and dentistry (what we were planning to do in the new school at Connecticut, and a tradition in some European countries). In both Scandinavia and Eastern Europe, I was able to observe working interprofessional teams, especially in dental and primary care clinics. I also was interested in the teaching of social and behavioral sciences in medical and dental education. Before coming back, I visited Great Britain, where social science research and teaching groups were very active. The journal *Social Science and Medicine* sponsored its first international Social Science and Medicine conference that year in Aberdeen, Scotland, with attendees from all over the world. I met most of the medical sociologists in Europe and continued contact with many of them, becoming a regular attendee at these conferences. A few people were calling for interprofessional teamwork in the delivery of health care and social services in Great Britain, but interprofessional education of students was largely impeded by the absence of intersecting educational pathways for the different health professions and occupations.

At that time, the British were beginning to probe the issue of interprofessional teamwork at the postgraduate level, and over the next 25 years the government and the National Health Service moved toward mandating such collaborative efforts. My return visit in 1982 resulted in my meeting a number of the IPP pioneers in Britain, including John Horder, John Fry, Barry Reedy, Katherine Elliott, Lisbeth Hockey, and Margot Jeffreys. I invited Barry Reedy to speak at the 1982 IHCTC conference, but when he was unable to attend, I gave a report of my sabbatical observations, entitled *The British are Coming*, in which I reviewed the rapid development and promise of both IPE and IPP in Great Britain.[22]

The frustrations of trying to publish the IHCTC papers and the inauguration of the modern *Journal of Interprofessional Care* in 1992 finally led Madeline (Mattie) Schmitt, a nurse sociologist at Rochester and host of the 1983 IHCTC, to contact Dr. Patrick Pietroni, editor-in-chief of the Journal, to tell him about the IHCTC conferences as a potential source of papers. In 1993, she was asked to join the Journal of Interprofessional Care Editorial Advisory Board, and the 17th IHCTC (1995) in Pittsburgh was attended by several British members of the Board, including Professor Hugh Barr. Hugh later became editor of the journal, as well as one of the most prolific thinkers and writers in the field, playing a leading role in every subsequent conference. Since then, Mattie also has been a leading voice for IPE and IPP both here and abroad.

Subsequent IPE conferences have included increasing numbers of colleagues from overseas. In 1997, the 19th IHCTC was held in London, in conjunction with the first international All Together, Better Health (ATBH) Conference with Mattie Schmitt and I serving as the two speakers from the United States. Since then, there have been five International ATBH Conferences, with attendees and presentations from a growing number of countries. In alternating years, there now have been three Collaborating Across Borders Conferences, celebrating mainly the IPE and IPP work going on in Canada and the United States. At the present time, IPE at the preprofessional and professional levels is alive and vibrant throughout Great Britain, the Scandinavian nations, and in a number of other countries around the globe.

Bud also was a pioneer in developing awareness in the US of the growing international interest and activity in interprofessional education and practice. When I had the opportunity to recommend the creation of a North American Division of the Journal of Interprofessional Care Advisory Board, he was my first choice, and the only physician. The Journal has been an important vehicle in making his seminal contributions to IPE visible internationally. As general editor, Hugh Barr worked with the publisher of the Journal to produce a Celebratory Supplement in 2007 honoring Bud, as well as to establish the annual Baldwin Award – first given in 2009.

—Madeline Schmitt, RN, PhD, FAAN Professor Emerita,
University of Rochester School of Nursing, Rochester, New York
(personal communication, January 18, 2012)

Meanwhile, in Canada

In the past decade, the IPE focus on this continent has shifted north to Canada, where one of the earliest IPE experiments occurred in the late 1960s, when John McCreary (a personal friend and mentor in the 1950s) invited George Szasz to explore and experiment with an interprofessional program for health professions students at the University of British Columbia.[23] Innovative and creative in concept and practice, there seems to have been insufficient time and formal structure as well as political support to ensure its survival.[24]

One of the attendees at the combined ATBH and IHCT conferences in the late 1990s was John Gilbert, who was named founding Principal of the College of Health Disciplines at the University of British Columbia in 2001. He was active in hosting the 2004 International All Together, Better Health II (ATBH II) Conference in Vancouver. Meanwhile, he and others persuaded the Canadian government to provide funding for the establishment of IPE and team training at a number of that nation's universities.

The first set of these grants were announced at the Canadian IPE conference held in Toronto in 2005, where Hugh Barr, John Gilbert, and I were keynote speakers. That same year, John invited me to the University of British Columbia as the McCreary Lecturer, where I found intense campus interest and activity and witnessed a creative, wildly enthusiastic, daylong competition between interprofessional teams of students. Since then, John has exerted international leadership in IPE and IPP at the World Health Organization, where together with Jean Yan, he initiated the global task force that produced the 2010 report, *Framework for Action in Interprofessional Education and Collaborative Practice*.[25] With ATBH III having been held again in London, ATBH IV in Stockholm, ATBH V in Sydney, Australia, and ATBH VI planned for Kobe, Japan, it seems clear that IPE has arrived internationally.

Where has the United States been in all of this?

While the United States has had a rather limited attendance at these international conferences until recently, the past decade in this country has featured a succession of national health care reports recommending interprofessional collaboration and teamwork as partial solutions to the many problems assailing our health care system. Despite these recommendations and the inherent logic of interprofessional education and practice, IPP and IPE have continued to languish, continuing a century-long "boom or bust" history.[26] Quite simply, there never has been an issue of sufficient medical and social power and importance to attract the kind of long-term, widespread professional, public, or governmental support needed to make IPE and IPP national priorities.

So what is different today? With a number of others, I believe that, for the first time, the issues of an overly costly, inefficient, and inequitable health care system and that of patient safety have emerged to command the attention of these major constituencies and to mandate improved communication, collaboration, and teamwork among the health professions. Additional good news is the recent publication of *Core Competencies for Interprofessional Collaborative Practice: A US Expert Panel Report*,[27] a report representing the collaborative efforts of six national health professions education associations.

The New Basic Sciences of Interprofessional Education

This mandate also takes form in the demand for changes in the education and preparation of all health professionals and has profound implications for IPE. For over a century, biomedical science has remained the standard knowledge base for medicine and medical education, as well as for the rest of the health professions. While this must continue, biomedical science has only a limited contribution to make in the solution of the many current social, political, and economic problems of patient safety and of the health care system. The new "sciences" required for understanding and solving these problems are basically those of the social and behavioral sciences: communication, collaboration, conflict management, consensus, role definition, decision making, and teamwork, as well as poverty, diversity, advocacy, and cultural, institutional, and organizational change. These are now center stage and will present new challenges for health professions education, as well as for the health care system.

My Other Passion: The Social and Behavioral Sciences

In the case of my long-term interest and effort to include the social and behavioral sciences in medical education, the story begins even earlier and, as with IPE, is still going on. I went to college intending to major in psychology, but found to my dismay that the department was totally disinterested in human and social behavior. After graduation, my plan to attend Divinity School was largely based on the fascinating work my parents were doing in ecumenism, and individual, group, and organizational dynamics.

Yale Divinity School didn't provide the spark either. But because of Yale's policy of allowing graduate students to take courses anywhere in the university, I discovered the Psychology Graduate Program across town next to the medical school at the Institute for Human Relations. In the spring of 1944, I attended what turns out to have been probably the earliest combined medical/social sciences seminar in the United States, conducted by Leo Simmons, a sociologist, and Eugen Kahn, a German-trained professor of psychiatry, with the participation of graduate students from a number of fields.[28] It was truly interprofessional and I loved it! At the end of the course, I asked Prof. Kahn where I could learn more about this kind of thing and he said, "Haf you effer considered medicine?" It was the last thing in my mind, but for my fieldwork that summer, I chose to serve as a student chaplain at the Massachusetts General Hospital. That experience was a turning point in my life. I was treated in such a mature, collegial manner that I decided that my desire to serve others could be better met in medicine than in the ministry.

Medical School

With its "graduate school" philosophy of education, Yale was probably the only medical school that would ever have tolerated me. Actually, I was lucky to get in. It was the only school I applied to, largely because I had a job and room and board on the college campus that I figured could pay my way through medical school. The first 2 years were not easy. After summers of learning experientially in my parents' international service-learning communities, the didactic learning of endless facts seemed meaningless, and I took full advantage of the "Yale System" to skip class and study on my own. Lucky for me, I had only to pass my National Board Exams to progress into the clinical years. Once there, the picture changed completely! Suddenly, learning was familiar and exciting again – experiential, problem-based, task-oriented, in small groups, with real responsibility, hands-on experience, and close teacher-learner relationships – I was back in my familiar learning environment. I fell in love with pediatrics and completed my residency training at the University of Minnesota and my fellowship back at Yale.

Starting Out

In 1952, I was planning to enter pediatric practice in California, but a boat trip up the Inner Passage off British Columbia made me fall in love with the Northwest. I was given 48 hours to make up my mind. As soon as we landed in Seattle, I made a call and by that evening, I had a job in the three-person Pediatric Department at the University of Washington's new medical school (how hiring practices have changed!). I don't think I've ever fully appreciated how lucky that decision was. Not only did it stimulate my interest in interprofessional practice and education, but also it reestablished my awareness of the relevance of the social and behavioral sciences to medical practice, as we dealt with and taught about family and social systems.

My assignment was to teach in the outpatient clinic at the Seattle Children's Hospital in the mornings and at the Child Health Center in the afternoons. The latter was funded by the Children's Bureau and involved a team of health professionals offering health maintenance services to the children of the WWII veterans attending the University. I thought I was in heaven! We had a truly interprofessional team, composed of two pediatricians, two nurses, a social worker, medical technician, dentist, dental hygienist, psychiatrist, and psychologist, each with our own students from the University. Since we offered basic courses in growth and development, as well as in child and family health and family dynamics, it wasn't long before we were teaching our students in concert – my first interprofessional teaching experience, and possibly one of the first consciously designed IPE experiences in the health field in this country.

When I left Seattle 5 years later, it was to take a child psychiatric residency in Boston, hoping to ensure my place as a clinician and teacher at the University of Washington, which was well on the way to becoming a research powerhouse, but had been unable to recruit a child psychiatrist. At the end of my training, however, the promised position in Washington did not materialize, so I accepted a position in pediatrics at the Children's Hospital at Harvard. Again, I was lucky enough to work at two sites, both with interprofessional teams and students. One was Harvard's Family Health center (which was very like my Seattle position and had superb research social scientists on staff). The other was the Forsyth Dental Research Institute, where I published my first paper on the interprofessional collaboration of dentist, nutritionist, hygienist, psychologist, and pediatrician.[29]

The Social and Behavioral Sciences in Dental and Medical Education

My research program (I had by now accepted the value of research) featured the application of theories and methods of the social and behavioral sciences to issues in dental health. Shortly, I was among the founders of an organization called Behavioral Scientists in Dental Research. It was at Forsyth that I established my first department of social and behavioral sciences in 1965. By 1967, I was on the planning committee for a new combined medical-dental school at the University of Connecticut, where the students would study together during their first 2 years. With ten funded positions, I assembled a unique group of people, each of whom had both clinical and social science degrees. Two years later, the scores of our students on the new National Board Part I exam in the Behavioral Sciences were among the highest in the country.

My interest in the social and behavioral sciences was further stimulated in 1969, when the National Institute of Child Health and Human Development funded a series of four National Invitational Conferences on "Behavioral Sciences and Medical Education" over a 2-year period, which were attended by 137 of the important social scientists and medical educators in the country.[30] Ten of us attended all four conferences and ended up founding the Association for the Behavioral Sciences and Medical Education. In the early 1970s, Association for the Behavioral Sciences and Medical Education meetings were held twice a year as medical schools established Departments of Behavioral Sciences and sought teachers who could prepare students for the newly required National Board of Medical Examiners (NBME) Part I examination in the Behavioral Sciences. In the beginning, partly reflecting the number of "orphan" subjects that had quietly begun "invading" the preclinical curriculum, the exam (and the new departments) also included such subjects as Biostatistics, Nutrition, Ethology, Ethics, Growth and Development, Human Sexuality, Death and Dying, and Health Care Systems.[6] In time, however, many of these topics were taken up by other departments and became established parts of the curriculum. In many ways, it was a confirmation of the frequent observation that it is evaluation that really drives the curriculum.

From 1976 to 1984 I served as a member and later chair of the NBME's Behavioral Sciences Test Committee. Unfortunately (in my view), in the early 1980s, in an effort to increase their purview, the Chairs of Departments of Psychiatry approached the NBME with the claim that "behavioral science" (note the loss of the "s") was really a "basic science" of psychiatry (ignoring the social sciences) and there was a virtual takeover of the examination, together with the addition of the term, Behavioral Science to their departmental titles (again without the "s"). Since then, there have been fewer social and behavioral scientists serving on the committee.[31]

> Without your efforts, the role of the behavioral sciences in medical education would be vastly different than it is today. Without the early inclusion of the behavioral sciences in the National Board Exams, students would not even be exposed to these essential concepts and ideas during their education. Without such exposure, the behavioral sciences would be less a part of medicine, and both patients and patient care would be poorer for the omission. Helping to define what is and should be a part of the conversation about medical education stands as one of your greatest contributions.
>
> —*Steven Daugherty, PhD, Longtime colleague and faculty member;*
> *Rush University Medical School, Chicago, Illinois*
> *(personal communication, January 30, 2012)*

The Social and Behavioral Sciences as Context and Perspective, Rather than Content

The long-delayed, greater acceptance of the place and contributions of the social and behavioral sciences in the medical and health sciences curriculum has undergone somewhat of a gratifying revival in the past few years, with important publications, such as *Improving Medical Education: Enhancing the Social and Behavioral Science Content of Medical School Curricula*,[32] and *Behavioral and Social Science Foundations for Future Physicians*.[33] Perhaps more important, the Association of American Medical Colleges has recently revised the Medical College Admission Test (MCAT) to include much more about the social and behavioral sciences, as well as about ethics, culture , gender, and socioeconomic factors.[34] (*See* our successful 1970s preprofessional, undergraduate program at Nevada described above!) Unfortunately, both of the reports and the test may be interpreted as focusing on social and behavioral sciences, primarily as content

– as a collection of scientific observations, facts or actions paralleling those of the other basic sciences. Instead, we should be recognizing that the distinctive contribution of the social and behavioral sciences consists of providing a context and a perspective for better understanding the problems of health and disease and health care delivery – problems not always amenable or necessarily commensurate with evidence-based science. The paradox haunting medical education is that science strives for certainty, while the practice of medicine is characterized by uncertainty. Dealing with this uncertainty requires the use of multiple perspectives and differing ways of looking at and thinking about the patient or problem. The biological sciences can be viewed as supplying some differing, though integrated scientific frameworks for understanding the patient. Social and behavioral sciences can do the same, although they engage different conceptual frameworks, principles, metaphors, and language, and different ways of measuring effectiveness.[35]

> Most of us seem to live our lives fitting into the institutional spaces around us. Only the exceptional person is able to remake those spaces and broaden the possibilities, not only for him or herself, but for others as well. It is truly amazing how your story is not just your own, but continues to echo in the lives of those you have touched. You have asked the interesting questions, were willing to follow wherever they led, and always managed to gather together the like-minded to share the journey. Sometimes the seeds planted take more than a lifetime, even an extraordinary lifetime, to grow. Those who have shared even part of the journey with you will never forget. You remind me always, not just where these ideas come from, but how they need to grow to make the future what it deserves to be.
>
> —*Steven Daugherty, PhD, Longtime colleague and coauthor;*
> *Rush Medical School, Chicago, Illinois*
> *(personal communication, January 30, 2012)*

Reflections

Common Ground: It's In the DNA

When I originally thought about the two educational innovations to which I have devoted most of my professional career: Modeling Interprofessional Education and Practice, and Introducing the Social and Behavioral Sciences into Medical Education, the idea of the Double Helix came to mind. What is clear to me today is that my two passions share a common DNA and are more completely intertwined and interactive than I had earlier realized. As I look at my career, much of the time, I've been working simultaneously or with one or the other, discovering, rather than always fully perceiving their vital and essential connection. The fact that both innovative efforts still remain to be fully realized after over half a century reinforces the importance of an expanded application of Kuhn's thesis; that efforts at transformative, innovative reform in fields other than science also require fundamental, paradigmatic shifts in conceptual thinking before they can be fully understood, realized, and accepted. Kuhn's[3] lesson for innovators may be that such paradigm shifts occur rarely and only after sufficient buildup of supportive thinking and experience enable such a paradigmatic shift to burst through the limitations of established ways of thinking and conceptualizing.

Lessons Learned

I've learned so much during the course of writing this chapter. Only as I was summing up did I realize the extraordinary confluence of people, events and experiences that seemed to make all this happen. I've been so lucky: lucky to have had the childhood experiences in diversity and travel; lucky to have had two parents who questioned the thinking of their day, advanced world-mindedness, internationalism, ecumenicism, culture and diversity, and developed adult, experiential, and service-learning methods for teaching and learning.

Indeed, it was only at the end of this manuscript that I also realized the powerful impact the World Health Organization's definition of health in 1948 had on me and the inception of my interest in IPE and IPP at the University of Washington's Child Health Center in 1952. The belief that "Health is a state of complete physical, mental and social well-being and not merely the absence of disease or infirmity" was a real game-changer for me and for many others. Such a "health model" brought about a paradigmatic shift in thinking about health and disease and the care of patients. It served to establish health care on a par conceptually and practically with the powerful, existing "disease model" of care, bringing all of the health professions into the picture as important and equal contributors to the care of patients and the maintenance of health in the community. As such, it empowered and liberated them to contribute and to collaborate in care and education in novel and creative ways. The Child Health Center accepted and operated completely within this new paradigm, setting in motion a lifelong personal and professional mission.

Innovators (like researchers) must accept living in unknown and unrealized spaces. The world of "what is yet to be" is emergent and unpredictable, where ancient mapmakers once warned mariners, "There be dragons here." Take courage from W.H. Murray's[36] statement from *The Scottish Himalaya Expedition* (and frequently attributed to Goethe) that "the moment one definitely commits oneself, then providence moves too."

Innovation in complex human systems like education – witness Maria

Montessori's radical ideas of early childhood education – seldom achieve easy or universal acceptance. Nature, especially human nature, reveals its secrets reluctantly. Learn to live with questions. Is it the right time, the right place? Are you ready? Are others ready? More important, is it the right thing to do? Patience with the process may prove to be the ultimate virtue. As Rilke[37] counseled in his *Letters to a Young Poet*, "Be patient toward all that is unsolved in your heart and try to love the questions themselves."

The Way of an Innovator

Having served on the faculties of eight medical schools, two dental schools, three graduate schools and two schools of social work, as well as a college President and on the staff of two major national medical organizations, there have been many moments when I (and others, I'm sure!) have wondered just what sort of path I was following. Frequently, it was not until I looked back at a particular experience that I realized how well placed and important it had been for me. A recent piece in the science section of the *New York Times* interviewing Eric Lander, Director of the Broad Institute at Harvard and Massachusetts Institute of Technology, gave me some insight into these questions. He said, "Biography is something of a confection. You live your life prospectively and tell your story retrospectively, so it looks like everything is converging."[38]

The Way It Is

There's a thread you follow. It goes among
things that change. But it doesn't change.
People wonder about what you are pursuing.
You have to explain about the thread.
But it is hard for others to see.
While you hold it you can't get lost.
Tragedies happen; people get hurt
or die; and you suffer and get old.
Nothing you do can stop time's unfolding.
You don't ever let go of the thread.

—*William Stafford*

Poetry usually goes right to the heart of such things. So, when I first read William Stafford's poem "The Way It Is,"[39] I experienced a real "mini-Satori." What a sense of enlightenment – intellectually, spiritually, even physically! Someone else really understood my life's puzzle. Why I had made the choices I did? Why I so often felt ill-equipped and uncertain about my decisions? Why I couldn't see the way forward at times? Did I always have to live through an experience before I understood it? If you don't read the poem, I think you will miss a lot of my process.

Now in my 90th year, I live with a lot of pain and limitation of movement. Spinal stenosis. I have resisted a cane until recently, and now it's a walker. The worst pain seems to be coming from the poor, tired, struggling muscles that seem to be trying to hold me up straight. But I have "miles to go before I sleep." I have a job. I go to work every day. I even get paid! I just got a raise!! The body may hurt, but the passion burns as brightly as ever. Besides, even now, my two particular passions have yet to be fully consummated. So I have to keep writing and contributing. Also, I'm still excited by life, and with my life. How could I not, when I have been so extraordinarily blessed with good luck and fortune – good health, a beautiful, resourceful, supportive spouse, a happy marriage (54 years!), a long life, intelligence, incredible opportunities and friends, as well as bright, creative, innovative, long-lived parents, who were way ahead of their time and whose ideas and work have extended far beyond them.

Parker Palmer has this concept of "living divided no more"; when your internal values and your external actions are resonant. Bud has always been an exemplar to me of living the "divided no more" life. He inspires me always, and I (and others) have joined his "community of congruence." Whenever we are together at AAMC [Association of American Medical Colleges] or ABSAME [Association for the Behavioral Sciences and Medical Education] or in Relationship-Centered activities, or on the phone, or even reading e-mails, there is a certain calmness that seems to come over us and a confidence that "everything will be OK." Bud's inner wisdom about interprofessional teamwork, the importance of the behavioral and social sciences, his rock solid goodness and values, plus his amazing life experiences make it a pleasure to just be with him. After all, we are human "BEings," who all too often get caught up in human "Doing." I love being in his "community of congruence."

—Joseph F. O'Donnell, MD, Associate Dean for Community Affairs,
and Professor of Geriatric Medicine, Dartmouth College Medical School
(personal communication, January 12, 2012)

References

1. Bloom SW. Structure and ideology in medical education: an analysis of resistance to change. *J Health Soc Behav.* 1988; **29**(4): 294–306.
2. Ludmerer KM. The history of calls for reform in graduate medical education and why we are still waiting for the right kind of change. *Acad Med.* 2012; **87**(1): 34–40.
3. Kuhn TS. *The Structure of Scientific Revolutions.* Chicago, IL: University of Chicago Press; 1962.
4. Association of American Medical Colleges. Physicians for the twenty-first century: report of the project panel on the general professional education of the physician and college preparation for medicine. *J Med Educ.* 1984; **59**(11 Pt. 2): 1–208.
5. Schofield JR. *New and Expanded Medical Schools, Mid-Century to the 1980s.* Washington, DC: Jossey-Bass; 1984.
6. Kennedy DA, Pattishall EG, Baldwin DC. *Medical Education and the Behavioral Sciences.* Baltimore, MD: Association for the Behavioral Sciences and Medical Education; 1983.
7. Kane RA. *Interprofessional Teamwork.* Syracuse, NY: Division of Continuing Education and Manpower Development, Syracuse University School of Social Work; 1975.
8. Baldwin DC Jr, Baldwin MA. Interdisciplinary education and health team training: a model for learning and service. In: Hunt AD, Weeks LE, editors. *Medical Education Since 1960: Marching to a Different Drummer.* East Lansing: Michigan State Foundation; 1979. pp. 190–221. Reprinted in *J Interprof Care.* 2007; **21**(Suppl. 1): S52–69.
9. Baldwin DC Jr, Baldwin MA, Edinberg MA, et al. A model for recruitment and service: the University of Nevada's summer preceptorships in Indian communities. *Public Health Rep.* 1980; **95**(1): 19–22. Reprinted in *J Interprof Care.* 2007; **21**(Suppl. 1): S70–5.
10. Dewey J. *Experience and Education.* New York, NY: Macmillan; 1951. (Originally published 1938.)
11. Stanton TK, Giles DE Jr, Cruz NI. *Service-Learning: A Movement's Pioneers Reflect on Its Origins, Practice, and Future.* San Francisco, CA: Jossey-Bass; 1999.
12. D'Avray L. Interview with DeWitt C. Baldwin Jr.: interview by Lynda D'Avray. *J Interprof Care.* 2007; **21**(Suppl. 1): S4–22.
13. Thornton BC, McCoy ED, Glover TW, et al. Interaction on health care teams. In: *Interdisciplinary Health Care Teams in Teaching and Practice: Proceedings of the First Annual Conference on Interdisciplinary Teams in Primary Care.* Reno: University of Nevada; 1980. pp. 201–15. Reprinted in *J Interprof Care.* 2007; **21**(Suppl. 1): S76–85.
14. Fisher BA, Hawes LC. An interact system model: generating a grounded theory of small groups. *Q J Speech.* 1971; **57**(4): 444–53.
15. Fisher BA, Drecksel L, Werbel W. Social Information Processing Analysis (SIPA): coding ongoing human communication. *Small Gr Behav.* 1979; **10**(1): 3–21.
16. Beckhard R. Organizational issues in the team delivery of comprehensive health care. *Milbank Mem Fund Q.* 1972; **50**(3): 287–316.
17. Rubin IM, Plovnick MS, Fry RE. *Improving the Coordination of Care: A Program for Health Team Development.* Cambridge, MA: Ballinger Publishing; 1975.
18. Wise H, Beckhard R, Rubin I, et al., editors. *Making Health Teams Work.* Cambridge, MA: Ballinger Publishing; 1974.
19. McGarvey MR, Mullan F, Sharfstein SS. A study in medical action: the student health organizations. *N Engl J Med.* 1968; **279**(2): 74–80.
20. Kindig D. Interdisciplinary education for primary health team delivery. *J Med Educ.* 1975; **50**(12 Pt. 2): 97–110.
21. Baldwin DC Jr, Rowley BD, editors. *Interdisciplinary Health Team Training: Proceedings of a Workshop.* Snowbird, Utah; 1976 September 6–8. Mimeographed. Distributed by Office of Interdisciplinary Programs, BHME, HRA, DHEW; 1978. Reprinted and reissued in 1982 by Center for Interdisciplinary Education, University of Kentucky, Lexington, Kentucky.

22. Baldwin DC Jr. The British are coming: some reflections on health care teams in Great Britain. In: Pisaneschi JI, editor. *Interdisciplinary Health Team Care: Proceedings of the Fourth Annual Conference*. Lexington, KY: Center for Interdisciplinary Education, University of Kentucky; 1982. pp. 3–17. Reprinted in *J Interprof Care*. 2007; **21**(Suppl. 1): S86–96.

23. Szasz G. Interprofessional education in the health sciences: a project conducted at the University of British Columbia. *Milbank Mem Fund Q*. 1969; **47**(4): 449–75.

24. Szasz G. Interview with George Szasz, CM, MD: interviewed by Lynda D'Avray. *J Interprof Care*. 2008; **22**(3): 309–16.

25. World Health Organization. *Framework for Action on Interprofessional Education and Collaborative Practice*. Geneva, Switzerland: World Health Organization; 2010. Available at: www.who.int/hrh/resources/framework_action/en/ (accessed September 11, 2012).

26. Baldwin DC Jr. Some historical notes on interdisciplinary and interprofessional education and practice in health care in the USA. *J Interprof Care*. 1996; **10**(2): 173–87. Reprinted in *J Interprof Care*. 2007; **21**(Suppl. 1): S23–37.

27. IECE Panel. *Core Competencies for Interprofessional Collaborative Practice: Report of an Expert Panel*. Washington, DC: Interprofessional Education Collaborative; 2011.

28. Bloom SW. *The Word as Scalpel: A History of Medical Sociology*. New York, NY: Oxford University Press; 2002.

29. Moorrees CF, Sisson WR, Peckos PS, *et al*. Need for collaboration of pediatrician and orthodontist. *Pediatrics*. 1962; **29**: 142–7.

30. Olmsted RW, Kennedy DA, editors. *Behavioral Sciences and Medical Education: A Report of Four Conferences*. DHEW publication no. (NIH) 72–41. Bethesda, MD: US National Institutes of Health; 1972.

31. Baldwin DC Jr. Some historical notes on the origins of the behavioral sciences and medical education in the United States: 1949–1987. *Ann Behav Sci Med Educ*. 2008; **14**(2): 72–80.

32. Institute of Medicine. *Improving Medical Education: Enhancing the Social and Behavioral Science Content of Medical School Curricula*. Washington, DC: National Academies Press; 2004. Available at: www.iom.edu/Reports/2004/Improving-Medical-Education-Enhancing-the-Behavioral-and-Social-Science-Content-of-Medical-School-Curricula.aspx (accessed September 11, 2012).

33. Association of American Medical Colleges. *Behavioral and Social Sciences Foundations for Future Physicians*. Washington, DC: Association of American Medical Colleges; 2011. Available at: www.aamc.org/download/271020/data/behavioralandsocialsciencefoundations forfuturephysicians.pdf (accessed September 11, 2012).

34. Rosenthal E. Pre-med's new priorities: heart and soul and social science. *New York Times*. 2012 Apr 15.

35. Baldwin DC Jr., Daugherty SR. The real contribution of the behavioral sciences: perspective, not content. *Academic Physician Scientist*. 2007; May 7–8.

36. Rilke RM. *Letters to a Young Poet*. London: Sidgwick & Jackson; 1945.

37. Murray WH. *The Scottish Himalaya Expedition*. London: J. M. Dent & Co.; 1951.

38. Kolata G. Broad Institute director finds power in numbers. *New York Times*. 2012 Jan 3.

39. Stafford WE. The way it is. In: *The Way It Is: New & Selected Poems*. Port Townsend, WA: Graywolf Press; 1999.

Concluding Reflections on Creating Enduring Change

Linda A. Headrick, Ann H. Cottingham,
and Debra K. Litzelman

OUR GOAL IN THIS BOOK WAS TO PRESENT A WEB OF STORIES FROM people whose work in health professional education touched the lives of others in important ways. After spending almost a year imagining the book, dreaming about who we might convince to share their stories, getting them to say "yes!" and nurturing those stories into chapters, we are thrilled by the result. These are the human stories behind some of the most influential work in health professions education over the past 4 decades. Without this book, these personal stories might never have been told. They all contain important lessons for others who hope to change health professional education for the good of the patients and communities their learners will serve.

With coaching from one of the book series editors, Dr. Thomas Inui, we took one more step to produce this closing chapter. As described in the Preface, we conducted interviews with chapter authors using a standardized set of appreciative inquiry questions. The themes that emerged across these interviews tell a story of their own.

Again and again we learned about education innovators whose *personal and professional formation* was marked by vision, motivation, and values from their families of origin. These innovators' life experiences made them aware of gaps between what was and what should have been. They had a *vision* of how to close those gaps that motivated them to *take the risks* inherent in change. None of them did this alone; all emphasized the importance of partnerships and *teamwork*. They were mindful of the *context and culture*, both internal to organizations in which they worked and external in the larger environment of health care and health professions education. Their *open-mindedness and genuine curiosity* nurtured their learning over time, continually changing and improving their work. This was particularly important to the *translation and spread* of their programs, even to international venues. Overall, their effect on others created a *legacy* that met and transcended their initial vision. In this chapter, we share some of what we've learned.

Personal and Professional Formation

> *I picked up the basic message from my dad that the world is a trust-worthy place and people can be trusted even though they don't always fulfill your trust 100% of the time. Better to lose a few bets than to . . . go through the world in a distrustful way.*
>
> —Parker Palmer

The educational innovators contributing to this volume described the important roles that family, colleagues, mentors, and life experiences played in their personal and professional development. This included the formation of their values, perspectives on teaching and learning, and professional direction.

Family

Family often served as an ongoing source of support for the authors, reminding them of their original goals when faced with challenges and helping them hold true to their vision. Many also credited family with a key role in the creation of their vision, both by instilling core values and demonstrating progressive ways of thinking about human relations and education.

Lived Values

The authors shared that many of the values later integral to their innovative work in education were modeled and learned within their families. The value of trust modeled by Parker Palmer's father, for example, became central to the methods of personal and professional formation Palmer developed, including the Circles of Trust. It also guided his approach to the program's expansion and his interactions with new program facilitators. Other authors identified appreciation of diversity, humility, respect for others, curiosity, and an orientation toward inquiry as values core to their approaches to teaching and learning that formed within the lived experience of family.

It is easy to see the link between a family that promoted diversity as a core value and an innovator who later created educational methods that used our "differences" as a resource, as in Inui's Relationship-Centered Care Immersion

Conferences. Also evident is the link between an early upbringing that promoted Kelley Skeff's humility and respect for others and his creation with Georgette Stratos of a program infused with respect and unconditional positive regard. In that context, participants were empowered to take risks that lead to powerful learning, like role-playing difficult situations in front of colleagues.

Models of Innovation

Some authors attributed the roots of their "new" directions in education to methods they had seen modeled by their parents. Inui described his efforts to change the relational culture of academic health centers as prefigured by the culture change work of his mother. She was a pacifist who led the international student exchange program in their community as a means to promote peace and a community leader who spearheaded efforts to desegregate the local YMCA.

DeWitt (Bud) Baldwin's parents similarly influenced his perspective on adult learning. Twice each summer his parents led small, international residential workshops for a period of 6 weeks that brought together students from diverse backgrounds and used Socratic, experiential and small group learning methods. Throughout his career, Baldwin worked to transfer what he learned during those summers into the very different world of traditional health professional education: "I brought the experience of my parents into my own work, which was vital. I knew if you treated students in a certain way they would be far more responsible than if you treated them the traditional way." His pioneering work at Nevada, characterized by an interprofessional team approach to teaching and learning, early and frequent clinical experiences, and an attitude of respect for learners echoed his parents' summer workshops.

Life Experiences

The authors identified particular life experiences as teachers, in organizations and as members of national professional groups as important to their personal and professional development. They also cited personal experiences in the Peace Corps; the Human Potential Growth Center in Big Sur, California; kayaking; and others.

Experiences as Teachers

For some authors, teaching students and residents in patient care provided the "aha moment" when the need to improve health professional education became suddenly very clear and very personal. Eric Holmboe described a third-year resident who was brave enough to admit that she did not feel comfortable with her heart exam skills, in part because she had never been observed by a member of the faculty. He was in the midst of efforts to improve the assessment of clinical skills in a residency program where direct observation by faculty was not yet routine. "It helped me to say I don't care if they haven't been doing this in this program as the norm. It is really important and it is my responsibility as an educator to do it." He recognized that accurate and robust assessment and remediation activities were integral to developing the essential clinical abilities necessary to provide good patient care.

Hal Williamson shared his "aha" experience with a senior resident at 3 a.m. While discussing a patient's upcoming discharge, he described to the resident all the workarounds she would need to do to ensure that the patient would get the right care. He assured her that when she completed her residency she would be working in a system more oriented toward addressing patient needs. The resident observed that Williamson must find the situation at his own institution very "embarrassing." He observed, "the truth is it wasn't embarrassing for me until that time. And I went home and I couldn't sleep for the rest of the night. After that I thought, okay, I should be embarrassed and there is really no reason why the patient-centeredness of an academic health center should be any less than the small health system that that resident is going to practice in." This experience highlighted for Williamson the impact of institutional culture on health professions education (as well as patient care) and the importance of creating a patient-centered culture in which the care exemplifies the values taught in the formal curriculum.

Experiences in Academic Health Centers

Authors underscored previous experiences in academic health centers as helping to form their areas of professional interest. Some authors were particularly influenced by the ways that values impacted the priorities and culture of their institutions. Authors shared that previous institutional experiences gave them the opportunity to learn "what works" in one environment and the confidence to try them out on a larger scale. For example, Inui described how after receiving resources to create the Department of Ambulatory Care and Prevention at a previous institution, he worked intentionally to form the department in a way that fostered a relational culture. When hard times hit the institution, he found that his department "not only survived, but thrived because they hung together and just dug in and recognized that there is very little we could control, but we could continue to do our work together excellently, and they did. That was a lesson." Inui took his experience with relational culture to a much larger scale when he co-led with Richard Frankel, Deb Litzelman, Ann Cottingham, and others the Relationship-Centered Care Initiative at the Indiana University School of Medicine, with the goal of developing a relational culture across the entire nine-campus academic health center of the second largest medical school in North America.

Experiences in National Organizations

Authors' experiences in national organizations also influenced their professional development. From the acquisition of specific skills to exposure to new educational methods to improved understanding of the national discussion in their areas of interest, authors reported that their work with national organizations informed what they did in health professions education and took their visions to a higher level. As Skeff shared, "I had the opportunity to be one of the main presenters at two major organizations, and from these experiences and collaborations I could get a sense of what the work could mean nationally."

Mentors

Like family members, mentors provided psychological support and motivation for the authors, reminding them that the work they were doing was worthwhile even as it was difficult. Mentors often were important teachers and thought partners in the development of innovative ideas and strategies, sharing insights that became core to the author's work in education. Holmboe noted that "Lou Pangaro taught me that evaluation equals educational professionalism," a lesson that became foundational to Holmboe's work. Mentors brought a history and breadth of experience to their relationships with mentees. They pointed out opportunities and alignments that the mentee may not have seen. They were credited with helping to guide the authors toward a path that aligned well with the author's interests. Skeff observed, "Mentors pushed me in directions I didn't even know I wanted to go."

Vision

> I was totally convinced that what we were doing was extremely important . . . for the medical school and medical students . . . I felt like I was doing it for the greater good.
>
> —William Branch

The authors in this volume reported that they were particularly driven in their innovative educational work by the desire to achieve something they felt was critically important, the right thing to do, and larger than themselves.

The Greater Good

A number of our authors specifically described their work as an effort to accomplish a "global interest" or achieve "the greater good." In describing conversations at the University of Missouri that led to the decision to place exemplary family and patient-centered care at the forefront of their mission, Williamson shared that "people were willing to think about what's in the global interest as opposed to their own personal interest or the interest of something they were a champion for." In the quote that introduces this section, William Branch used similar language to describe his motivation to develop the innovative small group Patient-Doctor courses at Harvard. Baldwin mirrored these comments when he observed, "Interprofessional teamwork and social behavioral sciences . . . were basically egalitarian, empowering and relational . . . so I knew no matter how hard it was, . . . we were on the right track . . . Believe it or not, I felt like I was trying to change the world." Other goals that authors named included improving student learning to provide better patient care, sharing novel, "game-changing" teaching methods and gaining for faculty and students the freedom to *invent what they need to be successful*.

The motivation to accomplish a larger vision was often coupled with a conscious decision to place that vision before self-interest. Multiple authors used the term *altruistic* or *egoless* to describe their approach to the work. An "egoless" orientation may have enabled authors to take risks with their work that they may not have otherwise. Branch described a feeling of being disinhibited and freed to do what he felt needed to be done without concern for its personal ramifications: "I had a very strong belief that what I was doing was basically altruistically good . . . I wasn't inhibited by my own personal feelings. I felt freed to put everything in to it to make it happen . . . it allowed me to speak out more, push harder, work harder, kind of like being a revolutionary, I think." Elizabeth Armstrong similarly described taking risks in her approach to education by inviting students to share in both the learning and teaching, requiring her to step *out of the center of the classroom*. Thomas Viggiano and other authors echoed Armstrong's philosophy, recognizing the importance of keeping the focus on student learning rather than the author's own teaching.

Commitment

Whether focused on professional responsibility, improving patient care, health professional education, institutional culture, or the world, these authors acknowledged that their commitment to a larger vision, a vision they felt was good or right, helped to drive them forward through the challenging task of creating something new. Amidst the institutional controversies about his new courses, Branch stayed fully "committed, I'm going to go ahead." Branch had "discovered there was a hunger for this [developing one's capacity for compassion, empathy, respect] among the students and the faculty that no one appreciated . . . this is so important we just have to move forward." These education leaders used their energy, commitment, and openness to help others participate in and more fully develop the capacity to carry on the work. Stratos described herself as having "a high level of innate enthusiasm. I think there's a lot of joy inside of me that I bring to the work . . . I feel like I can sustain a group of people who are putting themselves on the line, with high energy and patience to help them go through their journey during the training [at Stanford]."

Risk taking

They [faculty learners] have been welcomed into a community and welcomed in to a laboratory, and what they are going to be doing with us is experimenting. They are not going to hear what the right answer is.
—Elizabeth Armstrong

Risk in Innovation

Being an innovator entails risk. When doing something new, a good result is not guaranteed. Changes to tradition are rarely unchallenged. Most authors viewed risk taking as an expected element of innovation. They also saw it as an important ability to pass on to others.

Experiments

Some authors characterized their work as an "experiment" because there was no way to know beforehand whether the methods they were trying would be successful. In describing the development of the Moi University problem-based learning (PBL) curriculum, a learning method completely new to them, Haroun Mengech recognized that both faculty and students were "in an experiment." Faculty were not used to teaching in the PBL style, and students were not used to learning through a problem-based approach. It was not self-evident that the new approach would work. Armstrong shared her strategy for trying something new in the Harvard Macy courses: "We just run the experiment . . . and if we don't like it, if we get bad reviews on that particular exercise, we replace it for the next year." She freed herself and her colleagues to approach innovation confidently by explicitly limiting the impact of any change ("if we don't like it . . . we replace it for next year") and by framing the possibility of failure as an opportunity for learning.

Breaking with Tradition

Armstrong described the risk that innovators face: "From the outset we broke out of all the molds. We said it was going to be international. We said it was going to be interprofessional. In 1994 to bring those things up was totally an anomaly. I was challenged on every front . . . but I took the risk . . . At first they said only doctors and then I said, no, no, no we've got to have everybody who really works on teams . . . It's not about just the physician, it's the nurse in the room, the physical therapist in the room, the podiatrist in the room." Today education leaders consider interprofessional approaches to be essential elements of effective health care education.

Risky Hand-Offs

When a charismatic innovator is successful in developing and implementing a product there is always the question as to whether the same results can be reproduced by others. Palmer faced this risk when after 2 successful years he decided to expand his Courage to Teach work to different venues with new facilitators. He wondered: "What will happen if we meet at less luxurious retreat centers than the one where we ran the pilot program? What will happen as facilitators with different personalities and styles get in on the act? What if the group of teachers we work with are very different from those in the pilot group?" The decision to move the program forward was risky, but expansion was essential to accomplishing Palmer's larger goal of improving primary and secondary education (a goal which later grew to include health professional education and international venues) and was ultimately very successful.

Helping Others Take Risks

The authors described risk as an integral element of innovation; they felt that the abilities needed to take risk were important skills to foster. They used many different methods to prepare others to take risks in learning and innovation.

Safe Environment

Some focused on creating a "risk-free" environment that would provide a safe space for colleagues or learners to try new skills and instill the confidence necessary to take a chance on a new direction. Stratos described how the Stanford Program intentionally created this kind of setting: "Over and over again, I watch individuals . . . struggle with their own biases, revealing varying degrees of openness to new ideas. I see them gain confidence, security and open mindedness over the course of a month . . . At the end of the training they have become emissaries who feel prepared."

Authors shared that inviting learners and colleagues to speak up and share feedback created a space where they could take risks in their learning and innovation. At the University of Missouri, establishing a patient-centered culture for the whole system was predicated on establishing an organizational structure conducive to safe conversations. Williamson described the planning meetings at the University of Missouri as places where "people feel like the rest of the people in the room have the greater good in their head. They're not posturing, they're not representing a school, they're not representing a point of view, they're representing the whole health system and what is best for the whole health system . . . the safety part I think really has to do with people not feeling like they were being criticized . . . they felt like their ideas would be listened to and debated in a respectful way. And accepted for what they were."

Leveled Hierarchy

Leveling the traditional hierarchy was another risk-encouraging technique identified by several authors. Armstrong, for example, described developing name tags for participants that listed only name and institution, not titles, thereby intentionally creating a space that demonstrated from the first moment that *everyone is equal in the room.* Shirley Moore noted the value of both clinically- and research-focused nursing faculty participants in the Quality and Safety Education for Nursing (QSEN) initiative: "appreciative of the views and the importance of both roles, no hierarchy." Baldwin leveled the hierarchy among the health professional team in 1972 when he gave everyone – social workers, nurses, and physicians – the same salary on a Robert Wood Johnson Foundation grant. Fostering equality broke through social and professional norms of power to free learners and colleagues to take a lead, share ideas, become active participants in the learning process, and pursue a new and innovative direction.

Meaningful Work

In describing their own pursuit of innovation, our authors shared that working to achieve something that everyone found meaningful motivated them to take the risks necessary to make that innovation succeed. As Viggiano observed, "When somebody cares about doing something that is truly meaningful, they want to do it." Skeff and Stratos helped faculty participants both "reach back into themselves to become re-centered about who they are and simultaneously apply this deeper understanding by encouraging a process of ongoing inquiry and excitement about new ideas."

Communities of Inquiry

Many of our authors created communities of inquiry, inviting others to join in the process of discovery. Armstrong described this in her Harvard Macy work: "They [faculty learners] have been welcomed into a community and welcomed in to a laboratory and what they are going to be doing with us is experimenting. They are not going to hear what the right answer is . . . Many have not previously been asked to go to the balcony at their institution and look down and say, 'What could possibly be better here? How could we make the life of our students, the life of our patients better?'" Moore shared similar thoughts regarding her faculty colleagues: "We didn't need to have every faculty in every place be an expert; we needed to let them have a trial and error approach. We didn't come out with one approach that everyone needed to use."

Mengech explicitly instructed the Moi students that "We are going to facilitate the learning, but the learning process must come from you." The invitation to join as partners in discovery acknowledged that colleagues and students embarked on learning and innovation not empty of abilities, but with important prior knowledge and skills. It demonstrated respect and challenged others to take a risk, putting their abilities to work at a higher level. Baldwin used this approach in the new medical school at the University of Nevada: "The very first day they [the students] started medical school we trained them to take crisis calls in the community . . . We treated them as if they were already communicating; we just added to their communication skills. Most people teach interviewing skills as though the students have never done it before." Nevada's innovative program acknowledged and built upon the skills students brought with them, fostering confidence to take the risk of applying existing skills in a new context. Baldwin reported that when Nevada's early 2-year students transferred to other medical schools, they frequently graduated at the top of their new classes.

Broad Ownership

Authors also encouraged colleagues and learners to experiment by sharing ownership of the innovation. Viggiano said, "It was never my project. I submitted it as a Harvard Macy research project, and I worked on it quite a bit. But when you think of it this was really the faculty's and students' project. They owned this." Armstrong noted, "Those returning scholars [faculty who come back year after year to help teach the Harvard Macy course], who give the time, I would say basically freely, to teach with us for ten days, six days, whatever, feel in a sense, and rightly so, that this is their program."

By empowering colleagues and learners to take risks, become part of the experiment, and share ownership in the innovation, the authors fostered both innovation and leadership. Viggiano noted, "I like to think they [the students] emerged as leaders." Similarly, several of Baldwin's interprofessional education colleagues at Nevada earned doctoral degrees and became leaders at other institutions. Several of his students went on to become deans at institutions across the country.

Teamwork
• • • • • • • • • • • • • •

*If you get a group of good spirited people who want to do the right thing
and work at it over time, things actually do change.*

—Hal Williamson

All of the work described in this book was done by groups of people working in
teams. In each case there was clear and effective leadership, but the leaders were
quick to point out the importance of teamwork and the contributions of others.
They described how "at every step there was a group of us involved." They talked
about "the strength in union when people came together instead of working
separately" and the need to speak with a unified voice. Baldwin summed it up
when he said, "I didn't solve these problems. I enlisted people and these teams
solved these problems."

There also was joy in being part of a team that worked well together. Stratos
said, "It's really very wonderful when we can rely on each other to have our backs
that way." Moore described "a team of us who clicked . . . you fed off of the energy
and you gave a lot to it also . . . there was an affinity for the project, and we would
do hard work together and kind of play together."

Shared Goals

The leaders whose stories make up this book attracted people to work together
toward shared goals. Palmer reflected that, "I have always said that for me one
of the real markers of success in our work will be the number of such people
[serious-minded people who are doing heavy lifting in the world] we are able to
attract into our orbit and partner with in matters of mutual concern."

Often the invitation to join the work touched on core personal values. Skeff
described "a sense of being a part of something profound enough for somebody
to get back in touch with their initial mission, initial belief system, and initial
commitment to others." Viggiano was struck by how the complex problems they
faced were simplified "by focusing on learning, focusing on the commitment to
improve learning so that the students and the faculty could make Mayo Medical
School the best medical school it could be."

Effective Ways of Working

The stories in these chapters describe how people working together helped each
other, worked through conflict, and learned together. Armstrong described how
the Harvard Macy faculty developed and delivered courses that were noted for
their excellence: "the fact that we sit in on each other's sessions over the course

of the ten days or five days, whatever the program is, makes it not just manageable but very supportive. Our helping each other . . . thinking about how the different threads connect. Thinking about how the work of different people can link to each other." Moore told the story of a leadership team that developed a culture of honesty and promise-keeping: "definitely a culture of sharing, being honest, not being afraid of being provocative . . . We were again very quick to divide up tasks . . . okay you do this part, you do, you do, you do . . . you knew people were going to deliver."

All change involves conflict, and successful working groups deal with conflict effectively. Branch observed, "these kinds of activities that generate great passion . . . they almost predictively have conflict and schisms." Baldwin recalled, "We had such smart people. Occasionally we had a thorny person, but all of that was good because they challenged us." Reflecting on the QSEN movement as a whole, Moore described the challenge of bringing together the different types of nursing faculty who needed to be involved, ranging from those at the bedside to others entirely focused on research. "But we had this thread in common about change and the quality of care and doing it for better nursing . . . Some of this is the feeling of utter acceptance of each other's different approaches."

Inui described the benefits of working with "other individuals whom you respect from students to peers" and how important was the "willingness of the individuals who met regularly to just bring to the table in the most remarkably honest way what was happening to them." Learning with others was a major motivating force, even for those most would describe as "the experts." Holmboe said, "I love learning every time we do it [Faculty Development Course in Assessment] . . . I realize this is as much about my own professional growth as it is about me helping others."

Shared Credit and Pride

Sustainability depends in part on shared credit and pride. Regarding the success of the Patient-Doctor course, Branch remarked that there was "more credit to go around than there are people who take the credit for it." Reflecting on those who were part of establishing Moi University School of Medicine, Mengech described a "special relationship to those pioneers . . . the core group that came together in the beginning." Moore reflected on the power of writing together: "We did do a lot of writing along the way . . . that works on so many levels. It gets the word out in general, and it became a huge known project in nursing. But it also again builds team . . . and it builds pride."

Context and Culture
••••••••••••••••••••••••••

We simply got more in line with our cultural values and became more collaborative.

—Thomas Viggiano

The education leaders authoring chapters in this book were mindful of the context and culture of the institutions and external environments in which their work was embedded. They took advantage of the positives and mitigated the challenges.

Institutional Context

Leadership

Across the experiences described in this book, committed leadership clearly made a difference in moving new educational programs forward. At Moi University, the controversial PBL curriculum for the new medical school made progress because Mengech as the dean decided from the beginning that the school was going to take this direction. He described how the advertisements for faculty were written specifically for the new PBL curriculum at Moi.

Holmboe was able to introduce direct observation as a standard assessment method at Yale because "the program director, the department chair, the clinic director all understood the value and helped launch the program . . . their encouragement, understanding and [the] expectation from the program director" were very important to the success of the program. The leadership at Stanford provided strong support for an integrative approach between historically unlikely partners, in this case the School of Education and the School of Medicine. Skeff commented, "I was just fortunate to be at an institution that emphasized openness and encouragement to study another field at a time when it wasn't as commonplace as it is now and to attempt to integrate the lessons and principles of these two fields simultaneously."

Critical Mass

In several of the stories, a critical mass of like-minded individuals created synergy. Branch described how controversial doctor-patient courses were finally approved at Harvard because "the students got a petition and they argued strongly that this course should be made required. And many of the faculty did as well." Viggiano spoke about how he brought students and faculty together around the new curricular improvement program despite messages that "our faculty really thought that students didn't care." What mattered most was the students' "willingness to give us a chance to show them we did care about each other; we do want to help; we had just learned a way of doing things that made no sense at all." Moore talked about the importance of having five or six out of eight on their QSEN work team who had all participated in Paul Batalden's Health Professional Education Summer Symposium. She agreed that "this critical mass definitely influenced our culture of sharing, being honest, not being afraid of being provocative."

Existing Strengths

Many of the authors used existing strengths within their organizations as foundations to build on. For example, the Yale Internal Medicine residency had elements already in place that made it easier to build a new assessment program. Holmboe spoke about "an advisor system where every resident had an advisor they met with on a regular basis who also served as their clinic preceptor. It's a really nice system because you developed a good relationship with a core set of trainees . . . the foundation had been laid . . . to begin to move to enhancing the assessment component of the training program." Even with a strong curricular foundation, Holmboe faced challenges when introducing his direct observation assessment with individual learners. He sold the new program to current learners and to himself stating, "it wasn't necessarily a failure as individuals but a failure in the system. . . . I don't care if they haven't been doing this in this program as the norm. It is really . . . my responsibility as an educator to do it knowing that the only way to detect these deficiencies is that you have got to look and make sure the purpose was explained to the trainees."

External Factors

External factors such as the policies of accrediting bodies, external funding and congruity with existing trends also helped shape the direction of these new education programs. Stratos noted the enhanced dissemination of their clinical teaching program "when national accreditation bodies put more emphasis on faculty development requirements for residents and faculty."

Several authors mentioned the importance of receiving grants. External funding helped legitimize the innovators' work and opened up opportunities within their home institutions to implement and disseminate their ideas. Armstrong recollected, "it was money from the Macy foundation . . . that allowed me to feel I could experiment after I got all of the right permissions." The Robert Wood Johnson Foundation was instrumental in promoting Baldwin's pioneering work in the area of interprofessional education and the enormous changes in nursing education described by Moore. Similarly, Inui emphasized the importance of funding from the Fetzer Institute for the Relationship-Centered Care Initiative that affected both Indiana University School of Medicine and one-fifth of medical schools in Northern America. Moore summed up the recipients' careful shepherding of these monies: "we felt from the very beginning absolutely grateful for this money [from the Robert Wood Johnson Foundation] . . . resources were there and we felt the responsibility to spend them well."

Congruence with emerging trends lent a quality of serendipity to some of these efforts, a sense of being in the right place at the right time. Inui mentioned that the Relationship-Centered Care Initiative was like the "strumming of a cord that others could resonate with — we were a couple of years ahead of a wave of consciousness that maybe people would say was a good time to help teams [of medical educators and leaders from 25 schools of medicine] think about relational culture building." Clearly one of the earliest innovators in the area of interprofessional education (IPE), Baldwin spoke about "a fortuitous time of people, place and opportunity that made something possible . . . and I can't get away from the fact that the background of this [IPE work] was that it was in the 1970s and the whole country was on this liberalizing theme."

Open-Mindedness and Genuine Curiosity

I believed that one had to get into the river before you understand what kayaking was really about.

—DeWitt Baldwin

The innovators whose stories make up this book personally embodied learning, approaching their creative work with open-mindedness and genuine curiosity. They realized that no preparation could completely ready them to forge ahead with their "risky experiments." They jumped in and trusted that the process and the experience would shape the learning and the outcome. The authors also believed that their learners (whether students or faculty) were instrumental in co-learning and co-creating educational processes and programs. Although the authors built their educational programs on sound theory and an existing evidence base, they were not content to view their programs as complete but rather as evolving works-in-progress undergoing continual refinement.

Embodiment of Learning

After years of dedicated work building nationally and even internationally acclaimed educational programs, one might imagine the creators of these programs would carefully protect the value of their contributions. There is no doubt that the authors in this book wholly believed in the merit of their life's professional effort yet they were amazingly open to other people's perspectives and suggestions about their education innovations. They shared openly, listened, integrated the ideas of others into their work, and explored new venues in pursuit of ever-increasing excellence.

Stratos described herself as "someone who sees other people's perspectives and doesn't jump to conclusions, allowing them to express their point of view and be heard." Stratos went on to say that her open-minded stance has led to applying knowledge from one field to another, such as "applying the medical teaching to patient care interactions." Similarly Marcy Jackson described how Parker Palmer worked with a small group of facilitators to prepare them to "test" the model he'd developed, bringing "a groundedness and a confidence in the process . . . but also an openness and the willingness to learn from and with the group" as they expanded the Courage to Teach (CTT) work to include teachers in inner city schools participating in retreats in new regions of the country. Palmer recalled responding to one of the facilitator's questions: "well suppose we come back here . . . and we tell you it [CTT retreats] didn't work? What will you say then?" He remembered "just instantly, straight from my heart saying, 'Well, then I'll ask you what you want to try next.'" We all "did a lot of deep heartfelt learning together." Baldwin compared his long history of innovative work in IPE (experimenting with innovations 40 years before the most current wave of interest in IPE) to learning how to kayak, stating: "I believed that one had to get into the river before you understand what kayaking was really about. That's why I brought in the early clinical [experiences] and had pre-professional students in their sophomore year of college doing interviews with patients."

Respect for Learners

The authors respected learners and actively involved them in the learning process, teaching, and co-creating and improving programs. Mengech and others opened the second medical school in Kenya, Moi Faculty of Health Sciences (Moi) in 1990; Paul Ayuo joined in 1992. Establishing their highly controversial PBL curriculum, scrutinized closely by the Government of Kenya's Ministry of Education, was an exciting time of co-creating and co-learning among teachers and learners. Mengech, Moi's first dean, reflected "on the excitement as the staff and some students would go for weekends and critique the old [PBL] problems and come up with new ones or improve the old ones." Ayuo, Moi's current dean, continues to advocate for the merits of their PBL curriculum noting how "everyone [teachers and learners] in the circle is learning." Viggiano engaged learners to become critical members of medical education improvement processes by establishing his "golden rule" for improvement. Learners were "not just evaluating but . . . linking problem identification with solution generation."

Future Building

The authors' education innovations continue to morph to meet new needs. As we write this chapter, they are being exported to new and different types of learners. The authors collectively spoke about a commitment to excellence that places importance on staying receptive to the changing needs of the learners and learning environments. Holmboe made a promise to himself "to keep it fresh," noting the evolution of thinking in his program agendas over time. Armstrong spoke of "making the best possible program . . . to insure that the values are not only maintained but nurtured . . . to meet the new needs." Branch's expansion of the Human Dimensions of Medical Care Faculty Development program to a more diverse group of faculty provided important validation of the efficacy of his education innovations. He excitedly reported, "it really worked, it really worked for a bunch of people, not just for select people . . . we did this on a large scale."

An important measure of the value of an education program is the perform-ance of the graduates of these programs. Part of the 10-year review of the Moi School of Medicine was to interview the employers of the school's graduates. Ayuo was delighted to learn that the leaders within Kenya's Ministry of Health reported that "they could tell our grads apart from other universities" in the matur-ity of their clinical reasoning, decision making, and problem solving.

Translation and Spread

It doesn't seem to matter where we are . . . the human essence of what it means to teach other people seems to be a core value of everyone.
—Kelley Skeff

The growing success of the work of the authors led to opportunities and chal-lenges to expand their reach internationally. This prompted careful deliberations about whether the innovations would be relevant or adaptable to other cultures, and if so where and how. As they charted new waters, they readied themselves for resistance and even rejection of their carefully designed and tested education models and methods.

Global Impact

Several of the initiatives described in this book grew to substantial international footprints. Examples include the Harvard-Macy programs (Armstrong), Courage to Teach (Palmer and Jackson), and the Stanford Faculty Development program (Skeff and Stratos). The authors instinctively believed that much of their work would be exportable, yet they remained open to exploring and adapting during the process of internationalizing their programs. Concerns about limited resources, particularly the investment of time it would take to expand across continents, were considered in consultation with the authors' local trusted partners and advisors. Working in new countries was marked by the innovators' willingness to culturally adapt; they experienced relief and delight when underlying core principles and values held across cultures.

Jackson described their conscious decision making and analysis of needed resources before beginning the CTT work in Australia. Jackson felt "that this work [CTT] and how we do it and how we engage people in it has broad reach and possibilities and that we've got a lot to offer in various geographical places . . . but there was good conversation (with colleagues and board members) and we didn't just jump into this without thinking about what we might need for resources for the center and time and all of that . . . several people from Australia and Great Britain come to our gateway program for facilitator preparation with the desire to launch CTT in their country but they haven't had either enough experience or enough institutional help until recently." Once it was determined to expand CTT work in Australia, Jackson realized "there is a lot I don't know and can't know about bringing this into a new (international) context such as how diversity or privilege or social equity shows up differently in Australia . . . knowing that there is a lot that I don't know and can't know about bringing this into a new international context, I knew there was a lot of listening and learning that they would need me to do."

Core Principles and Values

In the process of global dissemination, the authors identified core principles and values that seemed to hold up across cultures. These emerged as archetypal patterns of how human beings teach, learn, and relate to one another.

With substantial experience in exporting the Stanford Faculty Development program, Skeff and Stratos have experienced the robustness of their clinical teaching theoretical framework and education methods across the globe. Skeff noted, "there is an international if not human orientation towards the helping of others that has become obvious regardless of where we are working with physicians, and it doesn't matter if it is the Far East or the Middle East . . . the international experience is largely a recognition and validation that the themes go across cultures. They probably reflect the commitment of people who believe in what they are about . . . the human essence of what it means to teach other people seems to be a core value of everyone." Similarly, Stratos observed: "the success I feel is that I see people embracing the role of being a helper of other teachers in such a deep, deep way – and it happens over and over and over again." Although earlier in their cross-cultural exportation of the CTT program, Jackson found there "is real robustness in the model and the philosophy behind their work and though there are many cultural differences in how they are manifest, the underlying roots and foundation are so accepted . . . and repeated patterns create the sense of a true archetypal pattern."

Legacy

This is not my program; it's not Harvard's program; it's their program; they own it and they feel responsible for maintaining a level of excellence.

—Elizabeth Armstrong

Over time, the authors built communities that spread the work far beyond what they might have achieved or even imagined on their own. Moore recalled standing in the midst of hundreds of nurse educators at a QSEN national meeting with a feeling of "all of them being part of the circle of contagion. They were all going to affect the place they worked, other faculty and all the students and it just felt like this huge influence. And also they were so positive about what this would do for health care, for nurses and how it would affect patients." Skeff described a sense of excitement about training second generation facilitators; that is "somebody who had taken our course from one of our trained facilitators [first generation] when they were a resident [and were] now enrolled in the Stanford [facilitator-training] course [themselves]."

Armstrong described how the Harvard Macy course alumni have stayed connected to the program, even returning to make their own contributions as teachers. They've told her: "'Liz, we have to keep doing this, we have to keep making it happen, we have to bring in our new colleagues. I want you to meet so and so because they would be wonderful faculty in this.' They come and take the course and then a year, 2 years, 5 years later they'll call or write and ask, 'Can I come back and teach again? Because we want to be part of growing this movement.'" Palmer described "creating a real sense of community among what's now 200 facilitators . . . by transmitting a shared culture and inviting people into a shared practice."

Many of the authors explicitly planned for spreading and sustaining their work. Regarding her decision to be part of the leadership of QSEN, Moore observed: "I think by starting with sustainability in mind it created a strong commitment . . . this was the time – this was the thing that was going to start the ball rolling that wasn't going to stop." Baldwin said he "learned to make connections at the heart. I would invite people to come and see us, to see what we were doing and they were glad to come." Branch remarked on the importance of moving his program to "a large scale . . . it really worked; it really worked for a bunch of people, not just for select people." He described the math related to spreading to other schools: "You talk about twenty-three schools. Let's just say we average nine people at each school. That's 200 people. That is a lot of people, and they can have a big influence."

Armstrong described her strategy thus: "If we want this to keep working, we have to keep improving. Making it the best possible program we can . . . innovative, role modeling . . . hope that the community will continue to support it, market it for us and bring their colleagues back . . . insure that the values are maintained, not only maintained but nurtured and even worked on to meet new needs."

Conclusion

The education innovators whose stories are told here are an inspiration to us as editors, colleagues, and friends. Their work has had an enormous impact, both within and beyond their home organizations. We hope that this book will spread that impact even further. We especially hope it speaks to readers early in their careers as educators who are wondering, "How is it possible that my dreams for the future might become real? This academic health center is so big, so complex."

Some of the answers to the question, "how is it possible?" can be found in this book and can be summarized as follows:

- stay true to your *values*
- commit to a *vision* that closes the gap between what is and what should be
- *take risks* with the help of partners
- nurture those partnerships through effective *teamwork*
- pay attention to the *context and culture* of the environment
- be *open-minded and curious* learners in a way that improves our work over time
- take advantage of opportunities to *translate and spread* your work to other venues
- invest in partnerships and build communities that can lead to a *legacy* of enduring change.

The stories we have collected in this volume tell us how we can live an undivided life both personally and professionally and at the same time create enduring education innovations that will shape and influence how medicine is practiced for generations to come.

Index

References to boxes, figures, photos and tables are in **bold**.

Index

Index

Index

Index

CPD with Radcliffe

You can now use a selection of our books to achieve CPD (Continuing Professional Development) points through directed reading.

We provide a free online form and downloadable certificate for your appraisal portfolio. Look for the CPD logo and register with us at: www.radcliffehealth.com/cpd

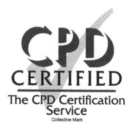

Milton Keynes UK
Ingram Content Group UK Ltd.
UKHW051924141024
449569UK00027B/1352